CONCERNING
THE ORIGIN
OF MALIGNANT
TUMOURS

CONCERNING THE ORIGIN OF MALIGNANT TUMOURS

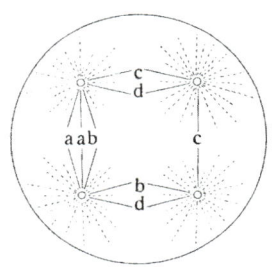

By

THEODOR BOVERI

Translated & annotated by

HENRY HARRIS

CONCERNING THE ORIGIN OF MALIGNANT TUMOURS

English Translation and Annotations Copyright © Henry Harris 2007
All rights reserved
Co-published in 2008 by The Company of Biologists Limited
     and Cold Spring Harbor Laboratory Press
Designed and typeset by Pete Jeffs, set in the typeface *Dolly* by Underware,
www.underware.nl

Printed in China

Library of Congress Cataloging-in-Publication Data

Boveri, Theodor, 1862-1915.
    [Zur Frage der Entstehung maligner Tumoren. English]
    Concerning the origin of malignant tumours / by Theodor Boveri ;
translated & annotated by Henry Harris.
        p. ; cm.
    ISBN 978-0-87969-788-4 (pbk. : alk. paper)
1. Cancer--Etiology. 2. Tumors--Etiology. I. Title.
    [DNLM: 1. Neoplasms--etiology. 2. Neoplasms--pathology. QZ 202 B783z
2007a]

    RC268.48.B6613 2007
    616.99'4--dc22

2007035051

A CIP catalogue record for this book is available from the British Library

10 9 8 7 6 5 4 3 2 1

Authorization to photocopy items for internal or personal use, or the internal or
personal use of specific clients, is granted by Cold Spring Harbor Laboratory
Press, provided that the appropriate fee is paid directly to the Copyright Clearance
Center (CCC). Write or call CCC at 222 Rosewood Drive, Danvers, MA 01923
(978-750-8400) for information about fees and regulations. Prior to photocopying
items for educational classroom use, contact CCC at the above address. Additional
information on CCC can be obtained at CCC Online at http://www.copyright.com/.

All Cold Spring Harbor Laboratory Press publications may be ordered directly
from ColdSpring Harbor Laboratory Press, 500 Sunnyside Blvd., Woodbury,
New York 11797-2924.Phone: 1-800-843-4388 in Continental U.S. and Canada.
All other locations: (516) 422-4100. FAX: (516) 422-4097. E-mail: cshpress@cshl.edu.
For a complete catalog of all Cold SpringHarbor Laboratory Press publications,
visit our World Wide Web Site http://www.cshlpress.com/.

Preface

Of the many biological monographs that appeared in Germany at the end of the nineteenth century and the beginning of the twentieth, very few are now remembered. Theodor Boveri's *Concerning the Origin of Malignant Tumours* is a remarkable exception. It is regularly quoted, misquoted and quoted out of context in our present day cancer research literature. That it should be quoted is in itself unsurprising, for it is one of the most prescient theoretical statements that the history of cancer research has produced. But why it should be so often misquoted is not so immediately obvious.

Boveri's monograph was published in Germany in 1914, the year that marked the outbreak of the First World War. He died a year later. His views on cancer had met a chilly response from the medical community, but it was not this that determined the silence that followed the appearance of his monograph. Its fate was mainly determined by the fact that the First World War and its ruinous aftermath for Germany effectively closed down biological research there for more than a decade. His previous monumental contributions to the study of chromosomes were well known to English-speaking scientists, but, given the lack of communication between England and Germany during the war years, it is understandable that there should be little evidence that many of them were acquainted with his theory of the origin of malignant tumours. Exploration of his ideas was no doubt also delayed by the inadequacy of the tumour chromosome preparations that could be made at that time.

As an act of piety, Marcella Boveri, his widow, who was an American, translated the monograph into English. Although Marcella's translation was not published until 1929, it is through this medium that scientists in England and America came to learn of Boveri's ideas about cancer. However, Marcella's translation has long been out of print and copies of the book are hard to come by. This probably explains why references to Boveri in the current English-language literature are often inept and obviously second-hand; young scientists rarely visit libraries these days.

The inaccessibility of the book led me to believe that it might serve some purpose if I were to produce a new translation of the German text, accurate I hope, and couched in a brand of English that does not repel the modern reader. I have also taken the liberty of appending extensive annotations, in which I have endeavoured, among other things, to show, with the acuity of hindsight of course, just how prophetic many of Boveri's ideas were.

Henry Harris
Spring 2006

CONCERNING THE ORIGIN OF MALIGNANT TUMOURS

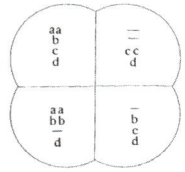

By Theodor Boveri

Professor at the
University of Würzburg

CONTENTS

I. Introduction

In the year 1902, I tacked onto the results of my experiments on the development of doubly fertilised sea urchin eggs the speculation that malignant tumours might be the consequence of a certain abnormal chromosome constitution, which in some circumstances can be generated by multipolar mitoses (Boveri, 1902). I had intended, even at that time, to put that assumption on a firmer footing in a separate article. But the scepticism with which my ideas were met when I discussed them with investigators who act as judges in this area induced me to abandon the project. I had to admit that a hypothesis in this field can be of value only if it leads to targeted new research and, above all, to new experimental investigations. And who ought it to be to decide to undertake such investigations if not the originator of the hypothesis himself? So, for some time now, I have carried out experiments that seemed to me to be relevant, admittedly without success so far, but my convictions on this score have nonetheless not been shattered.

It was the appearance of an article by O. Aichel (Aichel, 1911) that first prompted me to take the decision to communicate the hypothesis, and the evidence that supported it, in greater detail, even though I had essentially nothing more to offer than I had done ten years previously. To explain the origin of tumours, Aichel's article relies on facts that I had established in sea urchins and that gave rise to my own conception of tumours. But the hypothesis that multipolar mitoses might generate tumours is amalgamated by Aichel with his own view, published earlier, that the initial event in the generation of a malignant tumour is the fusion of a tissue cell with a leucocyte [1]. This notion casts the key elements of the hypothesis for which I am responsible in an essentially different light, so much so that it has become a matter of importance to me, now that my views have again become the subject of discussion, to set them out in their original form for readers familiar with the subject. But, in the end, I had another motive. The idea that there might be a connection between abnormal mitoses and malignant tumours has certainly cropped up often enough, but it has always been rejected, indeed so completely that in the recent literature it is curtly dismissed, if mentioned at all. The arguments that contradict the idea are easy to see. But one can nonetheless ask whether these objections are merely apparent and whether the more complete information that we now have about these chromosomal abnormalities might warrant, indeed necessitate, a reassessment of their connection with malignant tumours. What follows might serve as a stimulus to that end.

I write about this problem as a zoologist. I have no personal experience worth mentioning in any of the numerous specialised fields of tumour research. My knowledge comes almost exclusively from books. Given this, it is inevitable that I am unaware of many reports in the literature, that I overestimate the significance of many known facts and that I do not set enough store by others. But this article will doubtless contain even more serious defects, as is so often the case when an author makes an incursion into a field with which he is unfamiliar. You may well ask how anyone who has this to say about himself can hope to offer something worthwhile to investigators who have devoted years and even decades of work and thought to the tumour enigma. But there is one thing that has to be taken into account. The tumour problem is a cell problem [2] and, at the least, it is not impossible that a biologist who seeks to fathom certain phenomena in the living cell might be led to consider properties that cannot emerge from the study of tumours themselves but that nonetheless determine

1. This idea has recently been resurrected. It has been proposed that some of the characteristics of malignant cells such as invasiveness might be conferred on normally sessile tissue cells by their fusion *in vivo* with leucocytes. Fusion of tumour cells with polymorphonuclear leucocytes has not yet been described, but fusion with macrophages and lymphocytes has. It is commonly found that malignant tumours contain hybrids that have been formed by the fusion *in vivo* of the tumour cells with tissue cells of the host [Wiener, F. *et al.* (1972) *Nature New Biol.* 238, 155], but whether this phenomenon has any important role in determining the character of the tumour is not at all clear. Lines of mononucleate hybrids between macrophages and tumour cells have been established, and these continue to express macrophage markers *in vivo*. However, the hybrids isolated so far grow more slowly than the tumour cells themselves and are thus unlikely to be responsible for the progressive or metastatic character of the tumour formed.

their essential nature[3]. I ask that what follows be received with these considerations in mind.

I shall try to expound my thoughts in the briefest possible manner. I do not regard it as incumbent on me to measure my views against those of other authors. If my comments contain anything useful, it will be obvious without detailed discussion. There is only one author whom I need mention and that is David Hansemann[4], who long ago and on many occasions put forward ideas that are closely related to my own. Since his views on the significance of abnormal chromosome constitutions in the cells of malignant tumours have hardly been taken seriously, as far as I can see, what I have to say might seem doomed at the outset. Nonetheless, for all their similarity, there are such great differences, both in conception and in argumentation, between Hansemann's ideas and my own that the hypothesis I am now putting forward might perhaps contain precisely those elements that are missing in Hansemann's own.

Since no one will regard this essay as a source of information about the present state of tumour research, I shall cite only those contributions that workers in this field might not know about.

2. There are still some who contest this and in various forms advocate the view that the tumour problem is a 'tissue problem', not a 'cell problem'. By this they mean that the fundamental abnormality underlying the formation of a malignant tumour is to be found not in the genetic constitution of the malignant cells, but in the disruption of the organisation of the tissue in which the tumour arises.

3. Boveri, not having received a medical training, is very conscious of his position as an outsider. One cannot escape the impression that he must have met with a good deal of incomprehension from the medical fraternity. It is remarkable that his views on the origin of malignant tumours are guided almost entirely by his work on sea urchins and intestinal round worms.

4. David Hansemann (1858–1920), later ennobled as von Hansemann, is generally regarded as the originator of human cancer cytogenetics, although Hansemann himself acknowledges Hauser as a precursor. The chromosome counts that Hansemann made on mitotic figures in human cells fell far short of the actual number of chromosomes present, but he freely admitted the inadequacy of the techniques then available. He confirmed and extended the observations of several earlier workers who had noted the presence of abnormal mitotic figures in tumours, and he appears to have been the first to argue that the abnormal chromosome constitution produced by aberrant mitoses was an essential determinant of malignant tumorigenesis.

At this point I should like to express my warmest thanks to my former colleagues in Würzburg, Professor M. Borst in Munich, Professor R. Kretz in Vienna, and also to the present holder of the chair of pathological anatomy of our university, Professor M.B. Schmidt, for their many valuable suggestions.

The following observations on the essential nature of tumours seem to me to be best supported by the evidence. The cells of even the most malignant tumours can be formed from normal tissue cells. The determinants of this abnormal behaviour are to be found in the tumour cells themselves, not in their surroundings[5]. Although benign and malignant tumours have many properties in common, I have to agree with those authors who draw a sharp line between the two. In my view, there must be a fundamental difference between a tumour that grows in the same way as the tissue from which it is derived and one that does not. It seems to me that the transformation of a benign tumour into a malignant one, so often described, is a phenomenon of the same kind as the appearance of a malignant tumour at some site in normal tissue [6].

This statement does not cast doubt on the possibility that malignant tumours might sometimes arise from cells that are retarded in their histological differentiation (so-called 'immature' cells).

5. This is a further declaration of Boveri's position with respect to the two views discussed in Note 2. Theories that argue that malignancy arises not from an event or events taking place within the cell, but from disruption of tissue architecture, are sometimes referred to as 'field' theories [see, for example, Willis, R.A. (1948) *Pathology of Tumours*, Butterworth]. They have a long history, but have not found general acceptance in modern times because they do not account for the demonstrable clonality of many malignant tumours. Boveri, immersed in the study of chromosomes and guided by the belated flowering of Mendelian genetics, naturally assumes that malignancy, which is a heritable condition at the level of the cell, is determined by events that involve chromosomes, the carriers of the cell's heredity.

6. Here, Boveri confronts another problem for 'field' theorists: the stochastic nature of tumour formation. Boveri's own work on chromosomes, which is discussed in some detail later, leads him to conclude that the genesis of a malignant tumour is a rare cellular event. He is arguing here that when a benign tumour becomes malignant that change is again initiated by a rare cellular event within the benign tumour and not by wholesale transformation of a large number of benign cells.

But such cases seem to me to be exceptions compared with those in which the more pronounced independence of malignant cells is a secondary phenomenon determined by the loss of properties that were present at an earlier stage [7].

The essential elements of my point of view may therefore be summarised as follows. A malignant tumour cell is a cell with a specific defect; it has lost properties that a normal tissue cell retains [8]. In this respect, I am in complete agreement with the concept to which Hansemann has given the name 'anaplasia'. A cell in this drastically altered state reacts differently to its environment, and it is possible that this alone might account for its tendency to multiply without restraint. Such unrestrained proliferation is no doubt a very primitive property of cells [9]. Woodruff (Woodruff, 1913) has recently reported that, over a period of five years, he grew 3340 generations out of a single *Paramecium* under conditions where conjugation could not have taken place and without any special artificial stimulation. Woodruff has calculated

---

7. Boveri is not contending that differentiation and cell multiplication are mutually exclusive states, a primitive notion that sometimes sees the light of day even now. He is drawing a distinction between the possibility that a malignant tumour might grow out of a cell that is 'immature' for some other reason, and the idea that malignancy, caused by the deletion of some normal cellular component, might later incur a loss of specialised functions.

8. At this point, Boveri nails his colours to the mast: malignancy represents a loss of cell function, not the gain of a new function. The growth of the oncogene industry initiated more than half a century after the publication of Boveri's monograph was based on the assumption that oncogenes induce the gain of a new function that acts in a genetically dominant fashion. This view was strongly reinforced by the findings of tumour virology. Here, the assumption was that the virus, by introducing new genetic information into the cell, induces a new function that would also be expected to behave in a genetically dominant fashion. These views were, of course, incompatible with Boveri's insistence that malignancy was due to a loss of normal function. Experimental evidence in support of Boveri's position had to await the introduction in 1965 of cell fusion as a technique for studying the genetics of somatic cells. By means of this technique, it could be shown that normal cells contain genes that are able to suppress the malignant phenotype. Malignancy was thus seen to be a recessive and not a dominant character in the classical Mendelian sense and patently represented a loss of normal cellular function, not the gain of a new function. The discovery of genes that can suppress the growth of malignant tumours led eventually to the displacement of a sea of oncogenes by a tidal wave of tumour suppressor genes.

that if all the individuals in this culture had been kept alive, the amount of protoplasm generated from this one organism would have exceeded the mass of the planet earth by a factor of 10^{1000}.

It is only at the stage when the cells of solid tissues can be divided into those that merely propagate themselves and those that assume special functions that the latter stop multiplying exponentially. The cell ceases to be an egoistical entity and becomes an altruistic one, in the sense that it does not multiply except when the needs of the whole organism require it [10].

If now we regard the malignant cell as one that has lost certain properties and hence its normal reactivity to the rest of the body, then this change may well be enough to induce an altruistic cell to revert to its egoistical mode and thus release its multiplication from restraint. (Relapse of 'organotypic growth' to 'cytotypic growth', to use the picturesque terminology of R. Hertwig.) But it is also possible that, in the tissue cells of metazoa, special inhibitory mechanisms have developed that have to be eradicated before unrestrained multiplication can take place [11]. Be this as it may, both possibilities assume that elements present in the normal cell are missing in the malignant tumour cell. The following observations are an elaboration of this concept.

9. One way of looking at the multiplication of cells is that exponential multiplication and not 'rest' is the inherent steady state of all cells. As a consequence of evolution, all cells are so constituted that, given adequate nutrients and a clement environment, they will multiply exponentially without further stimulation. This idea evidently appeals to Boveri, who uses the data provided by Woodruff for dramatic effect. The key words are 'without artificial stimulation'. Boveri obviously believes, and so do I, that cells will go on multiplying of their own accord unless they are in some way restrained. There has been some controversy about the origin of this idea. It seems to have been first set down in print in the English-language literature in the 1950s, but it was apparently familiar to German biologists before the First World War.

10. This colourful anthropomorphic metaphor demonstrates once again that Boveri is not asserting that differentiated cells stop multiplying in metazoa, but that multiplication in metazoan cells is normally governed by the localised requirements of the body whereas malignant cells no longer recognise this form of control.

11. This formulation of the central idea gets even closer to the concept of tumour suppressor genes. Boveri envisages the existence of cellular mechanisms that normally exert a facultative control over cell multiplication and that are eliminated or impaired in malignant tumour cells.

II. Some observations from experimental cytology [12]

The thoughts briefly outlined in the preceding section give rise to the question: how can something be removed from a cell, and what are the consequences of such a deficit? Chemical and physical interventions may perhaps destroy certain cellular components without impairing the viability of the cell. I shall have something to say about such possibilities at a later stage. At this point, I am going to talk only about deficits created by the mechanical removal of parts of the cell. Fragments of cytoplasm can easily be removed from many kinds of cell, especially protists and egg cells. The numerous experiments that have been done to investigate this problem have, in general, reached the conclusion that in every bit of cytoplasm all the properties of the cytoplasm as a whole are latent, or, at least, that under the influence of the nucleus they can be regained. Any fragments taken from a protozoon, so long as they contain a nucleus, will regenerate complete animals, and nucleated fragments taken from eggs will produce normal embryos.

However, there are exceptions to this rule. In many kinds of egg, the process of differentiation is such that fragments taken from them generate fragments of embryos. Nonetheless, it is notable that, even in such cases, the cells that grow out of the egg fragment are not abnormal or sick. What happens is that the fragment can generate only certain sorts of cells. And even with eggs that behave in this way, the oocyte from which the egg is derived turns out to be totipotent. Nucleated oocyte fragments give rise to normal dwarf embryos.

---

12. This section is a dramatic illustration of just how much of an outsider Boveri was in the field of cancer research. The observations described in it were made entirely on sea urchin eggs, experimental material introduced by Oskar Hertwig (1849–1922) and exploited by Boveri with great virtuosity. It was on the analysis of sea urchin eggs that Boveri based his three great principles of chromosome behaviour: the individuality of chromosomes, their continuity from one cell generation to the next, and the different capacities of individual chromosomes to transmit heritable traits.

There is no reason to believe that tissue cells behave differently. Here too, a fragment containing a nucleus will retain the ability to regenerate the whole cell so that, in all probability, it is impossible – provided the cell survives the operation – to produce a permanent deficit in the cell by removing a bit of its cytoplasm.

In the case of the nucleus, similar experiments yield an entirely different result.

It is perhaps not inappropriate if, before discussing these experiments, I set out briefly the more recent findings concerning the structure of the resting nucleus and the contribution of the chromatin in somatic cells.

At fertilisation, two nuclei are brought together and (except in one particular respect that is of no interest to us in the present context) they are alike in the make-up of their chromatin. Not only do each of the two nuclei contain the same number of chromosomes but also, in favourable experimental material, it can be shown that, where a sperm contains chromosomes that have a characteristic size and shape, corresponding chromosomes of the same size and shape will be present in the egg. So one can draw the quite general conclusion that every chromosome in the sperm nucleus has its homologue in the egg nucleus.

Let us label the chromosomes in the one nucleus a, b, c and d. The other nucleus will also contain the same set, a, b, c and d. At fertilisation, the two *haploid* nuclei are amalgamated into one *diploid* nucleus, which now contains 2a, 2b, etc. Each chromosome in this duplicate set is then split into two, and a tightly controlled karyokinetic separation [13] of the daughter chromosomes ensures that a complete duplicate set is inherited by each of the two cells produced by the cleavage of the fertilised ovum. In the resultant resting nuclei, the individual chromosomes seem to break down. But we have every reason to believe that, within the stroma of the resting nucleus, every chromosome that contributes to the make-

---

13. Longitudinal splitting of the chromosomes and the details of karyokinesis were described by Walther Flemming in 1879 [Flemming, W. (1879) *Arch. f. mikr. Anat.* 16, 302]. The didactic exposition given here by Boveri would have been old hat for most biologists in 1914, but apparently doctors deeply immersed in the study of cancer needed it.

up of that nucleus continues to exist as a discrete region that reappears as the same 'chromosome' when the cell prepares to divide again. (Theory of the individuality of chromosomes.) In this way, the two sets of chromosomes amalgamated at fertilisation are inherited by all the cells of the individual. It is only in the germ cells that the so-called *reduction division* converts the duplicate set once more into a single set.

This symmetrical transmission of the chromosome constitution of the one-celled embryo to all the cells of the body is only possible if the mitotic figures are bipolar. If three or more poles take part in the mitosis – in the observations that follow we are going to assume that there are four poles – then the daughter cells will inherit an abnormal, and in its details an extremely variable, combination of chromosomes. The principal reason for this is that each chromosome can only split into two identical halves. Thus, if four poles are present, only two of the four daughter cells produced at the one time can receive the split product of any particular chromosome; the other daughter cells get nothing from that chromosome.

In addition to this, there is another important issue that must be taken into account. It is a matter of chance [14] which two of the four poles make contact with a particular chromosome, so that the four daughter cells not only have different chromosome numbers, but also have different chromosome combinations.

Let us assume, for diagrammatic purposes, that a cell contains eight chromosomes – 2a, 2b, 2c and 2d – and that it forms four poles instead of the normal two. One of the possible outcomes is shown in Fig. A. If we examine pole 1, we see that it makes contact with both chromosomes a, one chromosome b, one chromosome c and one chromosome d. From each of these chromosomes, pole 1 captures one of the two daughter chromosomes produced. The daughter cell formed around pole 1 thus receives the chromosome constitution 2a, b, c, d, as shown in Fig. B. In the same way, out of the configuration shown in Fig. A, each of the three other daughter cells will acquire the chromosome constitution shown in Fig. B.

14. A further affirmation of Boveri's conviction that cancer is initiated by a stochastic event.

It follows, first, that out of the same chromosome complement, a tetrapolar mitosis delivers a smaller number of chromosomes to the daughter cells than a bipolar mitosis: in our case, an average of four instead of eight. Second, it rarely happens that a daughter cell actually receives this average number; in general, some daughter cells get more than that and others get less. Third, it must happen that one or other of the daughter cells, and under some circumstances all four, fail to receive certain chromosomes. Thus, in our case, only daughter cell 1 contains a copy of each kind of chromosome: in cell 2, a and b are missing; in cell 3, a is missing; and, in cell 4, c is missing.

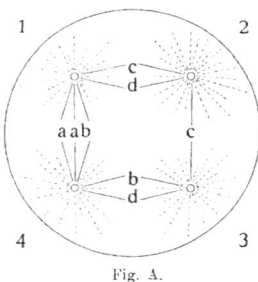

Fig. A.

In the foregoing case, the cell has a typical normal chromosome number but nonetheless has four poles. This does actually occur in nature and is probably a result of abnormal division of the centrosome.

The simplest way to produce a tetraploid mitosis is double fertilisation, which can be achieved in sea urchin eggs, for example, by adding very large amounts of sperm. Because each of the spermatozoa introduces one centrosphere that divides into two, four poles are formed. But these four poles are faced, not with a duplicate set of chromosomes, but with a triplicate set: one in the egg nucleus and one in each of the sperm nuclei. In this case, the chances that one of the four daughter cells might contain a copy of each kind of chromosome are much better.

Another way to generate tetrapolar mitosis is to suppress cell division in midstream. This can be done with eggs and blastomeres by pressing them together and shaking them. In this case, the two centrosomes and both groups of daughter chromosomes, instead of being allocated to two cells, are held together in the undivided mother cell and then proceed to form the new resting nucleus just as if cell division had been completed. When this composite double cell gets ready to divide, each of its duplicated pairs of chromosomes divides into two, and four poles are formed; but the nucleus now gives rise to four sets of chromosomes. As a result, each of the four daughter cells, formed at the one time, will

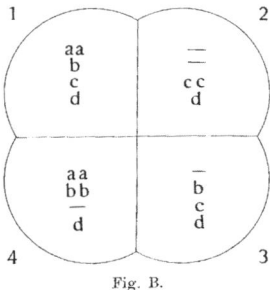

Fig. B.

receive, on average, the normal number of chromosomes, and the chances that at least one copy of each kind of chromosome will be present are again much better.

These observations are meant to show that, in multipolar mitoses, we have a means of achieving something that can otherwise hardly be done without collateral damage to the cell, namely the production of nuclei in which some parts are missing. And, in this way, we can answer the question that we posed in connection with the cytoplasm. What are the consequences of such a deficit in the case of the nucleus? To put the question more precisely: can a nucleus with a deficit of this kind regenerate what is missing and, if it cannot, can it remain viable without it?

The answer to the first question is that, as far as we know, even bits of chromosomes cannot be replaced. An abnormal chromosome number is inherited by all daughter cells provided that all subsequent mitoses are bipolar. The answer to the second question is that the overwhelming majority of cells with nuclei produced by multipolar mitosis are sick and perish[15].

To determine whether this ruinous effect that multipolar mitoses have is really a result of an abnormal combination of chromosomes, I have carried out a large number of experiments with doubly fertilised sea urchin eggs. I gave a short account of this work in 1902 and described it in detail in 1907 (Boveri, 1907)[16]. Here, my account of this work must be quite brief.

Three variants of dispermy can be distinguished in sea urchin eggs. We can call them the tetraaster type, the triaster type and the double spindle type.

· The tetraaster type is by far the most frequent. The two sperm nuclei unite with the egg nucleus. The four poles gather around this composite nucleus in a quadratic or tetrahedral fashion and, when the nucleus disintegrates, the equatorial plates are formed between the poles in the variable manner that I have described above.

· The triaster type can be produced artificially by shaking dispermic eggs vigorously shortly after fertilisation. In this way, the division of one of the centrosomes is suppressed in many eggs and, given the same chromosome constitution, only three poles are formed instead of the usual four.

· In the case of the double spindle variant, which is a rare aberration of the tetraaster type, only one of the sperm nuclei fuses with the egg nucleus; the other and its centrosome remain independent. Under these circumstances, two independent bipolar

15. This indicates that Boveri was well aware that aneuploidy was not in itself the precipitating cause of cancer, a confused view that one still sometimes hears today. Boveri regarded the chromosomal variability produced by aneuploidy as a mechanism that greatly increased the probability that cancer, a rare and stochastic event, might occur.

16. The paper referred to here is the last of the classical series begun in 1887. This work laid the foundation of our modern understanding of chromosome cytology.

spindles are formed, one containing the chromosomes of the egg nucleus together with those of one of the sperm nuclei, the other containing the chromosomes of the second sperm nucleus.

The developmental prospects of these three types of dispermy are very different. A dispermic egg with a double spindle, assuming that the egg divides into four, will generate one normal larva showing, at worst, a certain asymmetry. A dispermic egg of the triaster type generates, in addition to many completely pathological products, a number of partially or wholly normal embryos. Dispermic eggs of the tetraaster type, almost without exception, develop in a completely pathological manner; only a few partially normal larvae are found.

The first conclusion to be drawn from these differences in behaviour is that the three- or fourfold partitioning of the cytoplasm caused by dispermy cannot be responsible for the damage; for, if it were, no normal larvae at all would be produced by the dispermic egg. Nor can the differences we have described be explained by the abnormal chromosome numbers that the individual cells receive as a consequence of the multipolar mitosis. Furthermore, we know from experiments on merogony and partial fertilisation that eggs or parts of eggs containing as few as half the regular chromosome number can develop normally.

So, to explain the extremely variable outcome of double fertilisation, there is only one assumption left, namely that it is the wrong combination of chromosomes that makes dispermy so ruinous for the embryo. Put simply, the individual chromosomes must possess different properties such that only certain combinations permit the cell to function normally or, at least, keep it alive.

Both the egg nucleus and the sperm nucleus contain the right combination of chromosomes, which we have labelled a, b, c and d. This at once explains why, with a double spindle, the egg develops normally. For, in this case, two of the four primary blastomeres receive the derivatives of the normal nucleus of a fertilised egg; the other two receive the derivatives of a sperm nucleus.

The reason why, almost without exception, dispermic eggs of the tetraaster type develop into pathological forms is, in our view, because it is extremely unlikely that a tetrapolar mitosis would deliver at least one copy of all the different kinds of chromosome to each of the four primary blastomeres. With the same chromosome constitution and only three poles (the triaster type), the chances of this happening are appreciably better, which explains why one gets quite a few normal larvae from dispermic eggs of this type.

For further details and more substantial evidence, I must refer the reader to my specialist publications. In the last of these, in 1907, I remarked how closely the different ratio of normal to abnormal outcomes accords with the probability that the chromosomes are appropriately or inappropriately distributed [17]. I showed, moreover, that in many dispermic embryos only a proportion of the primary blastomeres generate pathological derivatives and the rest do not; this, on our assumption, is to be expected. Finally, I tried to justify the conclusion that, besides the chromosomes that are indispensable for the life of the cell, there appear to be some whose absence does not limit the viability of the cell, but only destroys or impairs other normal properties, for example the tendency to form connected epithelia or the capacity to stimulate the cells of another tissue [18].

The theory that different chromosomes have different capacities to transmit heritable traits, established in this way for sea urchins, has recently received decisive confirmation by the experiments of Baltzer (Baltzer, 1910) [19]. With certain interspecific crosses between different kinds of sea urchin, Baltzer was able to show that in the heterologous egg cytoplasm only four or five clearly distinct chromosomes derived from the sperm nucleus take part in the further development of the organism; the other

17. Boveri gives advance notice that his solution to the cancer problem will be a probabilistic one.

18. Here, he introduces the idea that chromosomal errors may give rise to defects in differentiation.

19. Fritz Baltzer was a pupil and later an assistant of Boveri. Almost half a century after Boveri's death, Baltzer wrote a devoted study of his life and work [Baltzer, F. (1962) *Theodor Boveri. Leben und Werk*, Wissenschaftliche Verlagsgesellschaft M.B.H.].

15 or 16 are excluded. This proves in a quite different way that there are qualitative differences between the chromosomes from the same nucleus.

The contents of this chapter can be summarised in the following way:

· All regions of the cytoplasm are composed of much the same sort of aggregated material so that every bit of it, if it is not too small, can regenerate the whole; the nucleus, by contrast, at least in *Echinus*, is made up of qualitatively different parts that cannot replace each other.

· These unique qualitatively different parts show up as discrete units in the mitotic chromosomes.

· If one ignores the sex chromosomes, every pronucleus contains all the chromosomes (probably one copy of each) that characterise the species.

· Only a cell that contains the complete set of chromosomes is normal; if some chromosomes are missing, the cell is in some way defective and, as a rule, perishes.

III. Relevance to the study of tumours

It is very likely that the findings set out in the preceding section on the nuclei of the sea urchin also hold true for vertebrates. We have long known that chromosomes of very different sizes are to be seen in the mitoses of vertebrates. Even if the experimental conditions are too obscure to allow us to discern a general rule, from what we have learnt with more favourable material, and in the light of the homology between animals and plants in these matters, we can hardly doubt the generality of what we have observed. This assumption is reinforced by the finding that a particularly striking chromosome or pair of chromosomes that have been detected in insects and nematodes, and which are connected with sex determination, can also be demonstrated in some vertebrates.

We may therefore regard it as probable that individual chromosomes have different properties in vertebrates too, and it is this assumption that forms the basis of the tumour hypothesis I have put forward. A malignant tumour cell is – and here again I take up the ideas of Hansemann – a cell with a specific abnormal chromosome constitution.

Although this assumption cannot be elaborated more precisely, there are some observations that might nonetheless be relevant. Estimates of the number of chromosomes in man vary widely. The mitotic figures illustrated by Winiwarter (Winiwarter, 1912) seem to show the best state of preservation. According to him, the diploid chromosome number in man is about 48 and the haploid number is therefore 24 (or 23)[*]. These 24 chromosomes must embody all the capacities inherent in chromatin. Now, if the

---

[*] So-called 'idiochromosomes' are formed, as first described by Guyer and then in an essentially different way by Winiwarter. According to Winiwarter, an idiochromosome is generated during spermatogenesis when one of the chromosomes fails to split into two and at the first cell division passes intact into one of the daughter cells. In this way, half of the spermatozoa formed have 23 chromosomes and half have 24 chromosomes[20].

20. In this footnote, Boveri keeps a straight face, but is obviously sceptical.

hereditary characters about which Mendel has taught us are located in the chromosomes, then each of the small number of 24 chromosomes must contain a large number of such units, most probably aligned along the chromosome in a specific order[21]. And if genetic experiments have demonstrated that in some cases certain properties are always linked together when they are inherited, these properties must, in our view, be represented in the same chromosome[22]. The manner in which red–green colour blindness is inherited is explained most simply if we suppose that the essential determinant of this defect is linked to the chromosome that Winiwarter regards as the sex chromosome.

So there is increasing evidence that specific segments of chromosomes are involved in every cellular event, whether we are dealing with properties that only become apparent in the cooperative behaviour of a larger complex of cells (e.g. in the shape of the liver) or properties determined by the presence and composition of cytoplasmic constituents (e.g. a pigment or a secretion). From this point it is but a short step to the concept that the intrinsic activity of the cell depends on the cooperation of specific chromosomal elements; this is precisely the conclusion that is best supported by the experiments on doubly fertilised sea urchin eggs.

Furthermore, these experiments on sea urchins have led me to conclude that there must be general properties that are common to all chromosomes and special properties that are limited to some only. It is probable, moreover, that many chromosomes are indispensable for the housekeeping functions of the cell and there are others whose absence might well impair the capabilities of the cell, perhaps even totally alter its character, but without making it sick.

If, in that case, the normal relationship of the cell to its surroundings is permanently disturbed, this, as I mentioned in my

21. This is a remarkably prophetic insight. As is well known, Mendel's celebrated 1865 paper was resurrected in 1900. In 1902, Boveri drew attention to the correspondence between the behaviour of Mendel's hereditary factors and that of the chromosomes, and he expounded this idea in greater detail a year later. To have suggested at that time that Mendel's units, which we now call genes, were arranged within the chromosome in a precise linear order was either a genuinely inspired guess or evidence of profound biological intuition.

22. Reduction of Mendelian linkage to the cytological level.

introduction, might in itself be enough to precipitate unrestricted multiplication of the cell and its progeny.

Another possibility is that there is a specific inhibitory mechanism in every normal cell that only permits cell division to take place when this mechanism is overcome by some special stimulus[23]. It would accord with our basic concept if one assumed that there were specific chromosomes that inhibited cell division. If their inhibitory effect were transitorily overcome, then cell division would resume. A tumour cell that proliferated without restraint would be generated if these 'inhibitory chromosomes' were eliminated[24]. In this case, the tumour cell would also lose all the attributes that were located exclusively in the same chromosome as the inhibitory factors.

However, the hypothesis that there are chromosomes that stimulate cell multiplication is also compatible with our proposal. In this view, cell division would take place when the operation of the stimulatory region of the chromatin, normally too weak, is enhanced by some active agent. The unrestrained proliferation of malignant tumour cells would then be due to a permanent excess of these stimulatory chromosomes[25]. This excess must, of course, be thought of as a relative matter. One might, for example, assume that the normal number for a haploid nucleus is one stimulatory

23. One modern view is that 'stimuli' to cell multiplication are merely agents that relax the inhibitory restraints normally imposed on all metazoan cells by the process of differentiation.

24. Very close to what was in fact found 55 years later when the suppression of malignancy was analysed by cell fusion. In these later experiments, it was found that the progressive growth of malignant cells was suppressed when they were fused with normal diploid cells, but it reappeared when certain specific chromosomes provided by the normal parent cell were eliminated from the hybrid cells.

25. Boveri feels obliged at this point to go through the gamut of other plausible possibilities, but he is clearly not enthusiastic about the idea that there are specific genes that stimulate cell multiplication. Indeed, the basic idea elaborated in his introduction to this monograph is that unrestrained proliferation is due to a loss or defect in normal cell function; and he is impressed by Woodruff's experiments with paramecia that demonstrate exponential multiplication over extremely long periods of time without any 'special artificial stimulation'.

chromosome and for a diploid nucleus two. If it should happen that, within an approximately normal chromosome number, there are three or four such chromosomes (an excess that can be produced by multipolar or asymmetrical mitosis), then unrestrained proliferation would result. But it is also conceivable that there could be a disturbance in the quantitative relationship of the stimulatory chromosomes to a single other chromosome.

I thought I should briefly mention these various possibilities. My own view is that the assumption that there is a specific inhibitory apparatus is less probable than the idea that the total chromosome complex of a tissue cell is so attuned to the influences of the rest of the body that, so long as there is no change in these influences, cell division is restrained. Cell division, it seems to me, takes place when a change in the environment has such an impact on the chromosome complex that it loses its customary equilibrium; but a disturbance of this equilibrium, and hence cell division, would also take place if a specific alteration in the composition of the chromatin occurred, which could be achieved by the loss of single chromosomes. And perhaps these might not have to be specific ones*. This interpretation, supported by the undoubted fact that tissue cells begin to multiply in response to different stimuli, seems to me to be more plausible than the assumption that there are specific inhibitory mechanisms. This would make it easier to explain the remarkably disparate rates of growth of malignant tumours. If there were a specific inhibitory organ in the nucleus, its elimina-

---

*If I assume here that the cells of malignant tumours multiply without restraint because they no longer respond appropriately to the environmental influences that normally hold back cell division, then one might suppose that essentially the same unrestrained proliferation might also occur in normal tissue cells if they are permanently withdrawn from the inhibitory influences of the rest of the body, provided of course that the nutrient supply is normal. The tremendous proliferation that takes place when fragments of tissue are cultivated outside the body, as described by Carrel, seems to favour this idea [26].

26. Here, again, the idea is that unrestrained cell multiplication is the natural propensity of all cells if there are adequate nutrients. In the case of tumour cells, the lesion they harbour is a loss of the ability to respond to the inhibitory stimuli of normal tissues. Normal cells retain this ability, but explantation from the body removes them mechanically from the influence of such stimuli.

tion would in all cases induce cell multiplication at the same rapid rate. If, on the other hand, we accept the possibility that proliferation is initiated by the elimination of different chromosomes, indeed no more perhaps than an abnormal chromosomal ratio, then one can understand how variation in the combination of chromosomes might account for all possible degrees of cell proliferation.

The foregoing observations lead us back to the question broached in the introduction to this essay, namely the relationship between benign and malignant tumours. The impression I have gathered from the accounts given in textbooks is, as I have already said, that there is a fundamental distinction between the two types of tumour. However, the essence of this distinction lies not in the division between benign and malignant characteristics, but in a boundary that is perhaps to be found elsewhere. The widespread conviction that the differences between the two are graded is, in itself, enough to warrant an enquiry into the question of whether the observations I have presented concerning malignant tumours also apply to benign ones. In terms of the hypothesis that there are chromosomes that inhibit cell division, one might see the distinction between the two types of tumour in the idea that in benign tumours these inhibitory chromosomes alone are eliminated, whereas in malignant tumours the combination of chromosomes in the rest of the chromatin also deviates from normality. An objection to this idea is that, in view of the small number of chromosomes, it is hardly plausible to make the extravagant assumption that there are chromosomes that act only as inhibitors of cell division. On the contrary, one might expect that the chromosomes in question also harbour other determinants whose abolition alters the character of the cell. A change of this kind does not seem to take place in benign tumours.

The other alternative is that unrestrained proliferation is due either to an excess or to a stable reinforcement of specific stimulatory chromosomes. Because this model does not entail the loss of any chromosome, it might explain the emergence of cells that differ from normal only in their potential to multiply and thus generate tumours that are benign. Malignant tumours would be defined by the fact that, in addition to having an excess of stimulatory chromosomes, they have lost certain other chromosomes.

What I have just said has provided a possible explanation for the genesis of benign tumours, but this possibility also exists in the concept I prefer; namely, that the propensity for sustained cell multiplication is simply due to a stable disturbance in the equilibrium of the chromosome complex. As above, the excessive proliferation could be explained by an excess of specific chromosomes, perhaps not even the same chromosomes in every case, but the dramatically abnormal properties of malignant tumours are then attributable to the concomitant loss of other chromosomes.

Although I must once again stress the purely hypothetical nature of the arguments I have advanced, mention must nonetheless be made of the fact that there are certainly links between the chromatin and the onset of cell division. In sea urchins, I was able to show in 1902 that too small an amount of chromatin relative to the amount of cytoplasm produces an intracellular stimulus to cell division that persists until further cell divisions re-establish a specified quantitative relationship between nucleus and cytoplasm (R. Hertwig's nucleocytoplasmic ratio).

I recently came upon another remarkable fact about sea urchin embryos. If, in experiments with interspecific crosses like those of Baltzer previously mentioned, one uses eggs that have been enucleated, one can get embryos with no more than four or five chromosomes (instead of 36–40). These embryos do not develop beyond the early blastula stage; but, before they perish, one often finds that the last mitoses are not bipolar but monopolar. This produces a so-called monoaster that cannot give rise to a cell division. So this too is evidence, albeit very indirect, that the composition of the chromatin is a decisive factor in determining whether the cell divides or not.

These instances are exceptional in that we are dealing in both cases with cells that cannot by the assimilation of nutrients regain the dimensions of the mother cells: each division reduces the size of the cell by half. This very fact precludes the direct application of these findings to the tumour problem. Nonetheless, they seem to me to be of some use in the analysis of this question. After the role of the centrosomes in the karyokinetic process had been clarified, we came very close to thinking that they governed the regulation of cell division. It was from them that the stimulus to division seemed to come. In the light of our present experiments, and especially those I have just described, the significance of centrosomes has been downgraded to that of tools that set up the mechanism that permits a cell to divide. But, in determining whether and how the cell uses this mechanism, the state of the chromatin, as I have explained, plays a decisive role[27]. It is therefore not improbable that every one of the stimuli that lead to cell multiplication operates through the chromatin[28]. And, if this is so, it seems possible that a certain stable change in the state of the chromatin might force a cell to divide again as soon as it is ready for it, as long as external factors such as inadequate nutrient supply do not impede it.

The main point of the observations that follow is not greatly affected by which of my more specialised assumptions concerning the dependence of sustained proliferation on the state of the chromatin one chooses to adopt. Abnormal mitoses can generate a host of different chromosome combinations so that, if our hypothesis is correct in principle, those combinations that make a cell a tumour cell must turn up occasionally, whether this is due merely to the absence of certain chromosomes or, in addition, to an excess of one sort of chromosome relative to the others. But, to stay with a unitary concept, we shall, unless some alternative is specifically mentioned, deal only with an absence of chromosomes (i.e. with a defect).

In the light of the foregoing discussion, I need hardly emphasise yet again that the essential element in my hypothesis is not the abnormal mitoses, but a particular abnormal composition of the

27. The relationship between nuclear genes and the centrosomes still remains largely obscure.

28. An early adumbration of the genetic operator model.

chromatin, irrespective of how it arises [29]. Any event that produces this chromatin composition would eventually generate a malignant tumour and can be considered tumorigenic: a disorder in certain chromosomes produced by a hereditary condition; destruction of chromosomes by intracellular parasites; damage of particular chromosomes by external agents that spare others; and other factors to which I shall come presently.

Nonetheless, I regard irregularities of mitosis as the usual way in which a nucleus of inappropriate composition is generated. I would like to say a few more words about this. So-called asymmetrical mitoses, which do not appear to be rare, may have much the same effect as multipolar mitoses. Asymmetrical mitoses, as the analysis of suitable material has shown, arise when the fibres associated with one of the two centrospheres do not form an attachment to all the chromosomes. The chromosomes that are attached to only one set of fibres – or, if division of the chromosome has already begun, the two unseparated daughter chromosomes – then pass to one of the daughter cells, whereas the other daughter cell remains devoid of these elements [30]. It is precisely these aberrations that can easily lead to a marked numerical excess of one type of chromosome relative to the others, if that is what is required.

Finally, as regards multipolar mitoses, these can take place in tissue cells in two ways. The first possibility is that, in the formation of the cell, the centrosome that it has received divides into three or four daughter centrosomes, instead of the usual two. To judge by the number of chromosomes present, I have seen cases of this sort rarely, if at all, in invertebrates. We do not know what causes the simultaneous multiple division of the centrosome. As certain injuries to this organelle impede its division, simultaneous multiple division might be due to some abnormal external influence, for which there is indeed some evidence.

29. Reiteration of the point made by Boveri earlier: aneuploidy is not the proximate cause of malignancy, but a karyological disorder that increases the chances of the proximate cause emerging.

30. A classical description of what we now call non-disjunction.

The second way that multipolar and, to be more precise, almost always tetrapolar mitoses can be formed is in the manner that I have already described, that is by the suppression of a cell division that is already underway. In both cases, it is generally found that one daughter cell is formed around each centrosome with its associated chromosomes. And, in both cases, these daughter cells, if they survive at all and provided no new abnormal event happens to them, multiply by binary fission from then on.

However, in another respect there is an important difference between cases in which multipolarity is produced by abnormal multiplication of the centrosomes and those produced by suppression of cell division. In the first case, a typical diploid chromosome set is divided up, that is there are initially two copies of each chromosome. On the other hand, when cell division is impeded, four copies result. It is clear that with the first of these two mechanisms there is a much slimmer chance that the daughter cells formed will contain copies of every chromosome in the set.

IV. The explanatory value of the hypothesis

Much of what has been found out about the origin and behaviour of tumours is neutral as far as my hypothesis is concerned; these findings are compatible with my hypothesis, but do not exclude other ideas. I will not go into this material but will limit my discussion to what, in my view, agrees particularly well with my position or seems to contradict it.

1. With the facts I described in Chapter II, I have tried to make it seem probable that if we regard a malignant cell as one that carries an irreparable defect, this defect is located in the nucleus, not the cytoplasm. Because this is the key point of my hypothesis, it is reasonable now to examine the relevance of this general principle to the tumour problem more closely, for one could object to the arguments I have put forward on the grounds that I have discussed only defects that are produced mechanically. It may well be true that you cannot produce a permanent defect by the mechanical removal of parts of the cytoplasm. Nonetheless, it has to be admitted that agents of a physical or chemical nature that act over longer periods might produce irreparable defects in the cytoplasm. And, indeed, certain specific facts that the study of tumours has revealed, such as the existence of cancers produced by X-rays or cancerous lesions simply called 'chemical' carcinomas, make it seem probable that the hypothetical defects in the tumour cells in these cases do not belong to the category with which I have been solely concerned.

I shall discuss later how I regard the origin of tumours that are produced by physical or chemical agents. Here, I simply wish to point out that it is, as far as I am aware, a generally acknowledged fact that carcinomas, for example, often arise at sites where abnormal physical or chemical influences can hardly be held responsible. If then the assumption is correct that a tumour cell arises because a defect has been produced in a hitherto normal cell, we do not need to involve complicated and long-lasting abnormal influences in order to produce this defect. But these considerations draw our attention to the simple abnormal divisions of both nucleus and cytoplasm produced in particular by multipolar mitoses. So it seems to me, given these completely spontaneous tumours [31], that the observations I made in Chapter II are still of importance in determining the origin of tumours. Having established there that mass deficits inflict permanent damage only on the nucleus, we have to assume that if the genesis of certain malignant tumours suggests that they harbour similar simple defects, then those defects, being irreparable, are nuclear defects.

2. If the aim of what follows is to illuminate generally acknowledged findings from the field of tumour research in the light of what we have already established, then I must first of all discuss one matter that has not been brought up anywhere else, as far as I know, although this matter strikes me as being of the greatest significance as regards the problem of malignancy.

It is very striking that, although different kinds of tumours can arise in the same tissue, each of these tumours typically has a unique character that is usually maintained in metastases and transplants. This phenomenon is no doubt due to the fact that, however dispersed a tumour might become, all its cells are derived from cells present when the tumour is first formed. If now

31. With the acuity of hindsight, it is easy to see that the notion of 'spontaneity' covers a multitude of sins. Nonetheless, in the conventional classification of malignant tumours, a sharp distinction is drawn between those that have a clear hereditary component in the Mendelian sense and those that have not. Despite Boveri's unitary view, or perhaps in ignorance of it, it was generally thought that the mechanism of carcinogenesis was different in the two cases. The 'two-hit' model adopted by Alfred Knudson brought the two together. He proposed, in 1971, that the same genetic locus was involved in both hereditary and sporadic cancers of the same kind. The argument, based on the epidemiology of hereditary and sporadic retinoblastomas, was that in the hereditary tumour one allele of the relevant gene is already deleted or inactivated in the germ line, so that to produce the malignant tumour all that is required is the inactivation or deletion of the other allele. But in the case of retinoblastomas that occur 'spontaneously', both alleles would have to be inactivated, which would explain the huge disparity between the incidence of the two forms of this cancer. The 'two-hit' model has run into some bothersome complexities, but it has swung opinion away from the view that the mechanism of carcinogenesis in hereditary cancers is fundamentally different from that in 'spontaneous' cancers.

one asks how the cells of the young, barely perceptible, primary tumours come to have their homogeneous character, the answer must again be that they go back to common ancestors that already had the same abnormal constitution. If one extrapolates further, one is bound to conclude that, in general, every tumour has its origin in a single cell.

This also accords with what is known about the very beginning of tumours. There seems to be unanimous agreement that, with extremely few exceptions, tumours do not arise as diffuse entities[32], but grow out of imperceptibly small origins. But then, if one's thoughts are forced to go back to a unit of the smallest possible size, there is no reason why the retrogression should be interrupted before one reaches the point where one can go backwards no further, that is, until one reaches a single cell.

However long it might yet take to prove this idea, I believe there is no escaping it; and I am convinced any theory of malignancy that does not take account of its unicellular origin is doomed.

The primordial tumorigenic cell, as I propose to call it in what follows, is, according to my hypothesis, a cell that harbours a specific faulty assembly of chromosomes as a consequence of an abnormal event. This is the main cause of the propensity for unrestrained proliferation that the primordial cell passes to its progeny so long as these continue to multiply by normal mitotic binary fission. But all the other abnormal properties that the tumour cell exhibits are also determined by the abnormal chromosome constitution of the primordial cell, and these properties will also be inherited by all the progeny of this cell so long as subsequent cell division takes place by normal bipolar mitosis.

If the assumption that every tumour is normally derived from a single cell is correct, this throws an interesting new light on the fact, stressed by all authors, that malignant tumours arise especially frequently at sites where there is chronic irritation.

32. Many pages of print have been published in support of the diametrically opposite view. For example, in 1967, Rupert Willis, an authority on the spread of cancer in the human body, published a textbook entitled *Pathology of Tumours* in which he argued at length that malignant tumours did not arise from single cells but from 'diffuse' lesions. Voices may still be heard proclaiming this doctrine.

I shall come back to this important observation in another connection; at this point, I should like to consider it from the following point of view. If the irritation was the immediate cause of the tumour, it would then be incomprehensible why tissues irritated uniformly over considerable distances do not undergo the same kind of transformation over the whole region or at least in many places within it. Chronic irritation obviously acts indirectly, which brings us very close to concluding that it gives rise to an inherently variable event that creates the conditions that generate a malignant cell in only a very small number of cases [33]. But the requirements of an event such as the one I am now proposing would be satisfied perfectly by abnormal mitoses.

3. On the strength of a whole series of investigations, it can be regarded as established that the histological modification of the tumour cell is accompanied by aberrant metabolism. Compared with what is made by the cells of the tissue of origin, it appears that normal products in changed proportions, or completely different products, are synthesised. One outcome of the altered metabolism is doubtless the frequent production of markedly different effects on the healthy surrounding tissue.

These facts agree very well with our hypothesis. The experiments on sea urchin eggs that I previously described have forced me to conclude that the individual chromosomes in the nucleus determine different metabolic reactions. If this is so, and if, in accor-

33. A restatement of Boveri's view of the significance of chromosomal disorder. Without wishing to enter into the philosophy of necessary and sufficient causes, it would, I believe, have been Boveri's position that aneuploidy is neither a necessary nor a sufficient cause of malignancy: not necessary because he does (reluctantly) admit the possibility that other mechanisms might also generate this phenotype; not sufficient because he repeatedly stresses that the chromosomal disorder in itself simply generates the variability that permits malignancy to emerge as a stochastic phenomenon. But he is convinced, nonetheless, that aneuploidy is by far the most common, albeit indirect, mechanism involved. Since almost a century of cytogenetic observation has confirmed that carcinoma cells are consistently aneuploid, Boveri's general thesis still stands. A recent claim [Hahn, W.C. *et al.* (1999) *Nature* 400, 464] that aneuploidy is not a precursor but a consequence of malignant growth has not been substantiated. At this point in his essay, Boveri returns to the question of 'indirectness'. How often might one expect that chromosomal disorder would engender a more immediate cause? This question is discussed in the section that follows.

dance with our hypothesis, tumour cells contain an abnormal assembly of chromosomes and hence produce an abnormal assembly of metabolites, then one can understand why the metabolism of such cells is also abnormal. A tumour cell that lacks certain chromosomes and has others in excess will produce many substances in excess and others in inadequate amounts, if at all. And it is very probable that, if the products of individual chromosomes, normal in themselves, interact at such aberrant concentrations, then the end products formed will be anything but normal. This would explain the altered effect that malignant cells have on their surroundings [34].

4. Our hypothesis does not predict how many different kinds of tumour can arise in any particular tissue. It is conceivable that for any one cell type there is one particular abnormal combination of chromosomes that endows the cell with the properties of malignancy, whereas all other combinations are harmless, or produce cells that are not viable, or produce cells that are viable but not capable of multiplication.

On the other hand, it is also possible that there are a number of different chromosome combinations [35] each of which confers a particular modification on the tumour. In terms of our hypothesis, this possibility seems most readily to accommodate the fact that, from one tissue, different malignant tumours may arise ranging from those that closely resemble the tissue of origin to those that appear to have lost the properties of the tissue of origin entirely. In the former case, in which the propensity for unrestrained multiplication is the only perceptible infirmity, perhaps only those chromosomes that govern cell multiplication are either missing or prevail. The more markedly the chromosome constitution deviates from normal, the less closely will the tumour resemble the tissue of origin, provided, of course, that the cells remain viable.

These deviations from normality in the constitution of the chromosomes do not necessarily mean that certain kinds of

34. The influence of cancer cells on their surroundings has now become a major area of investigation. But it remains largely obscure why certain cancers can destroy the afflicted individual long before the drastic symptomatology can be accounted for by the growth of the cancer itself.

chromosome are completely missing. Deviations could also arise if specific chromosomes present in the normal nucleus in two copies show substantial variation in copy number, as can happen for example when suppression of cell division generates a tetrapolar mitosis that may donate only one copy of a chromosome to one of the daughter cells and four to another.

In this connection, it is of interest that in plants (Œnothera)[36] it certainly looks as if a mere increase in chromosome number from diploid to tetraploid (i.e. every chromosome present in four copies) may generate a distinctly different kind of plant. With sea urchin eggs in which I induced tetraploidy artificially, I invariably obtained stunted larvae. How much more marked a change one would expect in the character of the cell if individual chromosomes were present in a variable number of copies!

If this factor really has the significance that we impart to it, then it would greatly improve the chances that secondary modifications would occur in the tumour cells. Be that as it may, with our present

35. A modern reader inundated in a sea of oncogenes might be surprised that Boveri does not envisage, or at least does not discuss, the possibility that lesions within the chromosome (mutations) might be involved in generating malignancy. But to be too surprised is to ignore the historical situation. The term 'mutation' was used by Hugo de Vries in 1901 to describe his finding that apparently new 'species' of plants could be generated suddenly from existing ones. Boveri was aware of de Vries's experiments, but like everyone else at that time he did not quite know what to make of them. After many years of general puzzlement, de Vries's results were found to be explicable in terms of chromosome mechanics and thus did not actually offer an alternative to Boveri's hypothesis. The term 'mutation' was given its modern connotation by Thomas Hunt Morgan whose first paper on the fruit fly *Drosophila* appeared in 1910. But the significance and world-wide acceptance of the work of Morgan and his associates Alfred Sturtevant and Calvin Bridges came slowly. Boveri's monograph appeared in 1914 and there is nothing in it that indicates that he was aware of the work of Morgan and his colleagues or at any rate appreciated its significance. Boveri died in 1915 and, despite failing health, worked to the end on experiments with enucleated sea urchin eggs. Analysis of the anatomical fine structure of the chromosome did not really begin until 1933 when Theophilus Painter, who at one time had worked with Boveri, discovered the giant chromosomes in the salivary glands of *Drosophila* [Painter, T.S. (1933) *Science* 78, 585].

36. This is the material (a primrose species) in which de Vries observed the phenomenon that he called 'mutation'.

knowledge, it is difficult to see a better explanation for the generation of different types of tumour from the one tissue of origin than that provided by our hypothesis. And that might well be seen as the weightiest argument in its favour.

5. In connection with the observations made in the preceding section, I should like to add a few words about the differences between the tumours of man and those of animals. Such differences have been emphasised by several authors: A. von Wassermann, for example, states 'a mouse tumour is not a human tumour'. In terms of our hypothesis, these differences could be due to differences in chromosome number. In man, as mentioned earlier, somatic cells appear to contain 48 chromosomes, whereas those of the mouse have only 32 [37]. By analogy with what one finds in invertebrates, these differences can be explained at least in part by the idea that chromosomes that are independent entities in one species are joined together in another. The basic chromosomal subunits will, in principle, correspond in the two mammals, so that their distribution in the individual human chromosomes must be different from that in the mouse chromosomes. In man, abnormal mitoses can generate combinations of chromosomal subunits that are impossible in the mouse, and perhaps also the other way round. This readily explains far-reaching differences between one animal and another in the tumours that arise in analogous tissues.

In general, we can say that the smaller the number of chromosomes a species has in which to accommodate the units of inheritance, the fewer different tumour modifications it can undergo, and the less chance there will be that a malignant tumour might arise; for the smaller the number of chromosomes in which the same units are accommodated, the more probable it is that the loss of even a single chromosome might remove genetic regions that are essential for the life of the cell. Indeed, it is conceivable that a species with a very low chromosome number might not be able to generate malignant tumours at all.

37. The diploid chromosome numbers given for the three animal species discussed in this section are, of course, incorrect, but that was the state of play at that time.

In the pig, the diploid chromosome number is said to be 20. It will be some sort of criterion for the validity of our hypothesis if, in this animal, malignant tumours arise less frequently than in man or more so, and it will also be relevant whether they are uniform or heterogeneous[38].

6. In the observations I have made so far, a malignant tumour is treated as a single unique event. But instances have been described, even if they are exceptional, in which several tumours of exactly the same type arise independently in the one organ or system. Indeed, there are instances in which a whole organ such as the stomach or the liver is riddled with cancers.

If we first consider merely the multiple origins of the tumour, this observation would not, of course, raise any difficulties for our hypothesis so long as one particular tissue could produce only one sort of tumour. One would assume that, within a more extensive area, abnormal mitoses occur so frequently that the combination of chromosomes required to produce a tumour would occur not only once, but often. All other combinations would not be noticed at all.

It is another matter if it is clear that the one tissue can generate malignant tumours with very disparate characteristics, each of which would, according to our hypothesis, be determined by a different combination of chromosomes. In these circumstances, the multiple independent production of precisely similar tumours would be inexplicable in terms of the mechanism I have advocated. For it is extremely improbable, if not inconceivable, that multipolar mitoses, in which the subsequent distribution of the chromosomes depends on chance, would give rise to multiple, and indeed numerous, daughter cells with exactly the same combination of chromosomes and never a combination that produces some different modification of the tumour.

38. The argument presented here will not carry much weight with a modern reader. There are obviously too many confounding factors – the life span of the different species of mammal, the rates of cell multiplication at comparable sites, the different conditions under which different mammals live out their lives, the hazards to which they are exposed, and so on – but the argument is of interest nonetheless, illustrating as it does Boveri's awareness of the problems raised by genetic linkage.

But even these cases do not, in principle, militate against our hypothesis. I have already mentioned Baltzer's finding in certain interspecific sea urchin crosses; namely, that of the 20 paternal chromosomes that the egg receives on fertilisation, only about four, doubtless specific ones, regularly take part in the mitoses. Their chromatids pass to the daughter cells in the proper way, whereas the other chromosomes do not divide at the right time and, depending on where they happen to be, are dragged off into one or other of the daughter cells. I have since been able to extend these observations by using, instead of intact eggs, enucleated egg fragments in which the fate of the paternal chromosomes in the foreign egg cytoplasm can be studied much more easily and followed into the later stages of development. The results of these experiments completely concur with the conclusions that Baltzer drew from his observations: it is a fact that only four (or five) of the paternal chromosomes regularly divide into two at mitosis. With certain exceptions that do not concern us here, their chromatids pass over into all the cells of the developing embryo and can still be demonstrated in the mitoses of the young blastula. The other chromosomes, depending on where they happen to be when the cell divides, either go to both daughter cells or only to one; thus, as cell division continues, the chromosomes are crowded into ever fewer cells, which sooner or later degenerate and are eliminated from the cluster. Embryos of this sort never make it beyond the young blastula stage. The cells with their four chromosomes sicken at almost the same time and shortly thereafter the embryo disintegrates*.

If an analogous event takes place in the tissues of mammals, this might perhaps provide an explanation for the problems with which we are here concerned, namely the multiple emergence of tumours of the same kind. It is well known that, among the mitotic disorders that one finds in tumours, there are also the so-called asymmetrical mitoses. These are bipolar mitoses in which only a certain number of chromosomes divide into two and are distributed in the proper way, whereas others are drawn to one pole with their two halves unseparated. This is a course of events

---

* I propose to communicate the details of this process elsewhere in the near future.

that corresponds very closely to the process in sea urchins, as I described a moment ago. If the chromosomes that behave abnormally in sea urchins are the same ones in all cases, rather than a random selection each time, then it is probable that the same holds true for the mammalian tissue in which asymmetrical mitoses occur. This leads to the following idea: let us suppose that for some unknown reason certain chromosomes develop an impairment in their connection to the process of mitosis and that this impairment is for the time being latent and is thus inherited by a large number of daughter cells. Then, the constitutional defect that these chromosomes carry can spread throughout a whole organ, indeed throughout the whole body, if it is already present in the egg[39]. Perhaps it is only with the onset of senescence that the hitherto latent defect manifests itself by the failure of these chromosomes to behave properly at mitosis. If so, wherever cell division takes place, daughter cells might be produced with specific recurring chromosomal defects. Should the chromosomes that fail to divide into two and thus pass undivided into a daughter cell be chromosomes whose absence turns a cell into a tumour cell, then the same sort of tumour could arise at numerous sites in the body; and organs in which cell division takes place constantly to replace worn-out elements could eventually be transformed into diffuse tumours.

Arising out of the particular situation that I have just described, there is yet another possibility that could be considered. If we ask what in interspecific sea urchin crosses determines the fact that some chromosomes divide in the normal way whereas others behave atypically, then the answer is the foreign cytoplasm. In our state of total ignorance concerning the composition of the cyto-

39. This idea, without invoking 'mutation' in its current sense, nonetheless foreshadows the 'two-hit' model, which I have already discussed. Boveri is proposing that a heritable genetic lesion may already be present in the egg and hence be transmitted to all the cells of the body, but the phenotypic effects of this lesion remain latent until a second event occurs. Boveri, of course, recognises the stochastic character of this second event, but seeks to explain the age incidence of most cancers by suggesting, hesitantly, that the onset of senescence might at the level of the cell favour the conversion of a latent defect into an overt one.

plasm, we do not know what that means. Nonetheless, we can say, in general terms, that a specific change in the surrounding cytoplasm has a detrimental effect on certain chromosomes but not on others*. But that makes it conceivable that a particular abnormal condition of the cytoplasm might be responsible for the production of a tumour. Furthermore, it does not appear impossible that a change of this sort in the cytoplasm might be determined by an external influence. If so, one cannot reject the idea that diffuse carcinomas, for example those of the stomach lining, might be elicited by external influences that produce a cytoplasmic change in the epithelial cells.

And, at this point, there is yet another possibility that must be considered. In these instances of diffuse cancerous degeneration, if it should be the case that the putative elimination of certain chromosomes is determined by a particular change in the cytoplasm of the cells, then perhaps the onset of the disease does not have to await the occurrence of mitoses at all. Baltzer, in experiments other than the ones on interspecific crosses that I have mentioned more than once, found that diseased parts of the chromatin can be eliminated from the nuclei of resting cells; if the right chromosomes are eliminated in this way, then that might make the cells malignant without more ado.

There is yet another analogy that might help to explain the multiple occurrence of one and the same kind of tumour. We know that there are animal genera that include species composed entirely of males or entirely of females. In these species, it appears that there is either a mosaicism of the gonads in which male and female elements are brought together, as is seen occasionally in carp for example, or, as in the case of the so-called 'hermaphrodite' bees, the whole body is a more or less complex mosaic of male and female regions. In many of these cases, the situation can be described as the dissemination of male regions within the female

---

* It may well be a task for future investigators to set up experiments with favourable material to see whether individual chromosomes can be affected by chemical means [40].

40. Another prophetic insight.

body, which brings us back to our own problem; for, in a similar way, cancerous regions with corresponding characteristics may be embedded at various sites in a healthy body.

We know from cytological observations that in many, if not most, animals the circumstance that decides whether the egg develops into a female or a male is whether the nuclei of the cells in the new individual contain or lack one or more specific chromosomes. It is therefore highly likely that the mosaic nature of hermaphrodites is to be explained by the fact that, within an embryo originally meant to become a female, asymmetrical mitoses occur sooner or later with the result that one of the daughter cells fails to receive certain chromosomes that in a normal mitosis it would have received. Such cells generate male regions, whereas the rest generate female ones. So there can hardly be any doubt that the factor that I have held to be responsible for the multiple occurrence of identical tumours, namely the elimination of specific chromosomes, is indeed responsible for the analogous production of certain hermaphroditic malformations.

What I have said will suffice to show that, in the interpretation of those rare cases of tumour formation that I have been discussing, we have the support of far-reaching analogies.

7. To what I have just said I should like to add an observation concerning the heritability of tumours. It is clear from the outset that, in the light of our hypothesis, heritable transmission can only exist in the sense that a particular predisposition is transmitted. It would indeed suffice if, in many individuals, the surrounding tissue found it much more difficult to suppress the emerging tumours than was the case in other individuals and if that property were heritable. But even the specific assumptions that our hypothesis makes do not exclude the possibility that it is a predisposition that is heritable. Thus, for example, diminished cellular resistance to influences that hold back cell division, and therefore lead to multipolar mitoses, might be heritable; and so might a tendency of the centrosomes to undergo simultaneous multiple divisions. Finally, the impairment of certain chromosomes, which I proposed in the previous section as an explanation for certain phenomena, might also be heritable. To complement what I have

already said, I would like to look into this last possibility more closely. If an impairment of particular chromosomes can occur in such a way that, here and there, perhaps under the influence of cellular senescence, they do not split properly during karyokinesis, both homologues in the diploid chromosome set would have to be impaired in the same way for a tumour to be produced[41]. Only if this is the case is there any chance that from time to time a daughter cell would be formed in which all the relevant chromosomes are missing. This idea assumes that the two homologous chromosomes have the same defect in both parental gametes. And that is how we reach the conclusion that the frequency with which tumours produced in this way occur is markedly increased by inbreeding. The fact that inbreeding does have such an effect appears to emerge from several different observations. I need only refer to *xeroderma pigmentosum*, which appears frequently in Jewish families and especially in marriages between close relatives, to put the heritability of the predisposition beyond doubt. It would be very interesting, whenever the opportunity to carry out such studies presents itself, to examine as carefully as possible not only the genealogy of the affected individual but also the histological characteristics of the tumours that arise.

8. It is not infrequently found that tumours arising out of one and the same tissue are composed of two or more different cell types. Our hypothesis can easily account for these too. If multipolar mitoses occur, the cell from which the tumour originates could simultaneously produce daughter cells that would contain different combinations of chromosomes, yet combinations that induce each of the cells to form a tumour. Thus, it appears possible that, from the very beginning, two or three more or less amalgamated tumours of different type grow side by side.

It is also possible that, in one of the cells of what was originally a unitary tumour, multipolar or asymmetrical mitoses occur and once again alter the initial chromosomal abnormality without extinguishing the viability of the cell or its capacity to proliferate without restraint.

41. This conclusion predicts pretty accurately what was actually found in cell fusion studies more than half a century later and is entirely consistent with the 'two-hit' model.

I believe that it is in this way that you have to explain the fact that, on repeated transplantation, a tumour cell line might separate into two or more sublines that may differ markedly from each other and from the original cell line.

What I have just said seems to me to make it fundamentally wrong to classify as a single tumour a complex tumorous growth that exhibits a diverse structure at different sites. Provided this diversity is not due to the response of the cells to different environments, one must recognise that there are as many tumours as there are cell types, even if under certain circumstances they mingle and form dense patchworks.

9. It seems to be generally accepted that the production of metastases is intimately connected with the effect that tumour cells have on their immediate environment. If the change in the environment results from an alteration in cellular metabolism, as our hypothesis postulates, then the hypothesis has already done enough to help us understand metastasis.

Nonetheless, I should like to draw your attention at this point to an interesting parallel between malignant tumours and the embryos produced by simultaneous multiple division in a doubly fertilised sea urchin egg. It is said to be especially characteristic of many tumours that their cells have a marked tendency to relax or altogether unloosen the normally tight structure of the tissues, an effect that probably makes a substantial contribution to the production of metastases. Something rather like that often occurs in the blastulae that grow out of dispermic sea urchin eggs. Normally the cells of the blastula form a monolayer of epithelial cells that are geared to close any gaps that might be formed and in this way restore the contiguity of the monolayer. But the cells in the blastulae of dispermic embryos frequently lose this capacity altogether. Although they show no reduction in their vitality or, at least, can undergo typical, even exceedingly vigorous cell multiplication, the blastula cells generated by the primary blastomere very soon lose their epithelial contiguity and form irregular, loose, friable heaps of spherical cells that have a microscopic appearance strikingly similar to that of a 'medullary carcinoma'.

We know from the investigations of C. Herbst (Herbst, 1900) that the blastomeres of sea urchin embryos round up and become detached from each other in calcium-free seawater. This means that, to form a cohesive epithelium, at least one specific substance is essential. By analogy with the aforementioned findings in dispermic embryos, one cannot fail to draw the conclusion that the normal nucleus determines the production of the substance that is required to maintain the cohesion of the blastula cells. If the chromosomes that specify this substance are missing, the cells lose their cohesiveness. The same assumption can be made about tumour cells that behave in a similar fashion.

10. Apart from changes in malignant tumours that apparently occur suddenly without transitional stages and which, according to our hypothesis, are caused by an additional change in an already abnormal chromosome combination, there seem to be others in which the character of a tumour changes gradually. These gradual changes may be present in the original tumours or first become apparent in the metastases, or, most tellingly, in the secondary tumours formed on transplantation. The reaction of the healthy neighbouring tissue to the presence of the tumour cells might be implicated in this phenomenon[42]. But it is also conceivable that the creation of certain abnormal chromosome combinations so perturbs the equilibrium within the nucleus that particular chromosomes go on changing under the influence of changes in other chromosomes. One group of chromosomes might eventually preponderate and perhaps even suppress the activity of others. It is therefore understandable that a malignant tumour that is at first closely similar to its tissue of origin progressively becomes less so and eventually becomes completely unrecognisable.

But one could also imagine that the exact opposite might be the case in certain respects. An inappropriate combination of

---

42. The relationship between a malignant tumour cell and its immediate surroundings, or, as the traditional metaphor puts it, the relationship between 'seed and soil', has long occupied the minds and engaged the emotions of countless investigators, and it has generated many theories of varying plausibility. Boveri can hardly avoid an occasional reference to the role that the extracellular environment might play in determining the behaviour of a malignant tumour, but he does not (perhaps cannot) go into this complex subject in any depth. He returns promptly to the role played by the chromosomes.

chromosomes might impair cellular functions profoundly from the very beginning, and later there might nonetheless be some measure of recovery, although not a return to normal. For example, it could happen that the preponderance of one kind of chromosome over another kind restricts the anabolic activity of the cell, but the subordinated chromosomes might undergo reactive hypertrophy and thus redress the balance.

Considerations of this sort make it plausible that a change in the character of a tumour might be only transient and might later be neutralised so that the original character of the tumour is restored. A few more words on this subject: earlier, I described the relationship between nucleus and cytoplasm as a form of symbiosis in that the individual chromosomes colonise the cytoplasm as independent entities. The chromosome cycle makes this comparison acceptable. These little bodies behave like protists, and it is conceivable that the transient inactive phases that have been observed in motile protists, whatever their cause might be, could also affect the individual chromosomes embedded in their cytoplasm. This inactivity might perhaps involve a single chromosome and impair its function. The result would be a change in the character of the cell during the period of inactivity. One might object that such periods of inactivity in individual chromosomes and the consequences that flow from them should also occur in normal tissues, for which we have no evidence; but tumour cells have certain peculiarities that favour the occurrence of such phenomena. First, in a nucleus that is abnormally constituted – and here we touch on a factor that we have already considered – the conditions under which the individual chromosomes operate differ from those present in normal cells. And second, one must remember that a normal cell has two copies of every chromosome, so that the suppression of one of them might pass unnoticed; by contrast, the cells of every malignant tumour have chromosomes present in only one copy and the suppression of this copy would then result in a temporary loss of certain cellular functions.

11. Given the significance that we attribute to the chromosomes, there is no escaping the conclusion that the differences between the cells of different tissues are ultimately determined by differ-

ences in the state of the chromosomes. These differences should not be envisaged as variability in the chromosome composition of different tissues, for we know, at least in certain cases, that different tissues have the same number of chromosomes. The differences we are talking about must be due to the fact that in every tissue certain parts of the chromosomes are greatly reinforced whereas in other tissues these same parts recede into the background or completely atrophy(43). This is not an idle speculation. Not only does the size and shape of the chromosomes appear to differ in different tissues, but we also know that there are cases where, in the process of differentiation, the original chromosome constitution of the cell actually evolves in two different directions. For example, in some species of *Ascaris*, heteropolarity of the cytoplasm results in the production of two different daughters from the one cell. One of the daughter cells maintains the original chromosome constitution, whereas in the other the ends of each chromosome are discarded and degenerate.

If the findings I have discussed justify my analysis of differentiation in various tissues, then these ideas might perhaps shed some light on certain observations that have been made in research on cancers. It is said that the cells of many malignant tumours undergo changes that make them resemble the cells of another tissue more closely than those of the tissue from which they originated. In terms of the ideas I have just been discussing, this is

---

43. Boveri is well aware of the fact that the regulatory events that determine differentiation cannot be changes in the number of chromosomes contained by cells of different tissues. On the contrary, the evidence at that time indicated that for any one species the diploid chromosome number was more or less the same in all normal somatic tissues. This meant that differentiation, if mediated by the chromosomes, had to involve changes in different regions of the chromosome. But differential expression of structurally unaltered regions does not cross Boveri's mind. No doubt 1914 was much too early for that. Boveri proposes instead that the enhanced or diminished effect of specific chromosomal regions is determined by changes in their structure. What the exact nature of these structural changes might be is difficult to decipher, for the terms Boveri uses to describe them are rather vague. They seem to suggest a gamut of regional amplification ranging from complete atrophy to gross hypertrophy. The 'puffs' in the giant salivary chromosomes of *Drosophila* come to mind.

understandable. If, for example, a tissue owes one of its special properties to the circumstance that certain parts of specific chromosomes in it are particularly well developed, whereas these same regions are rudimentary in tissues that do not express this property, then the elimination of the well-developed chromosomes by abnormal mitosis might result in a deficit that makes the cells look like those of another tissue.

12. However much opinions might differ about the causes of tumours, there is unanimity about the fact that malignant newgrowths occur especially often where a tissue is exposed to noxious agents.

Two further possibilities must be distinguished at this point. The noxious agents might act as chronic irritants, so that the tumour arises out of a background of inflammatory tissue rather like an abscess or some such thing; or a single transitory injury might in certain circumstances eventually give rise to a malignant tumour. Our hypothesis provides evidence for both these possibilities.

If for the time being we concentrate on the second alternative, that is, cases in which a blow or a crush injury, a burn or an excessive drop in temperature, are held to be the cause of a malignant newgrowth, then there is a striking analogy in the experiments on eggs and blastomeres. Here, squeezing, vigorous shaking, or excessive heat or cold can inhibit cell division without impairing the viability of the cells, so that the next time the cells propose to divide, a tetrapolar mitosis is formed with all the damaging consequences that this entails. Is it going too far to assume that the same influences might affect tissue cells in the process of cell division and, by inhibiting the complete partitioning of the cytoplasm, give rise to tetraploid cells? To be sure, to produce an abnormal chromosome constitution, the tetraploid cell must again undergo division. This takes place in blastomeres without further ado, for they have inherited an impulse to multiply from the egg. In tissue cells, however, an additional stimulus to cell division is required [44]. In healthy tissue, this may be long delayed or might never occur. One would therefore have to assume that the generation of a malignant tumour as a result of injury takes place in two stages that may be separated from each other by a lengthy interval. The first stage would be the inhibition of cytoplasmic partitioning due to an insult that occurs when the cell is in the process of dividing. This produces the tetraploidy. The second step, however, would be a stimulus that induces the tetraploid cell to divide by multipolar mitosis.

This idea might perhaps provide an explanation for certain specific observations that have been made in the field of tumour research. It has frequently been noted that carcinomas of the skin arise in scars, especially scars resulting from burns, that the scars are often present long before the carcinoma develops and that injury to the scar strongly favours the emergence of the tumour. The relevance of what I have said to cases of this sort is obvious.

The same may well be true for disseminated embryonic tissue, where it can perhaps be assumed that cell multiplication ceases because the normal parallelism between the nuclear cycle and the centrosome cycle has been disturbed, a parallelism that is essential for the production of a bipolar mitosis. In this way, large numbers of cells may be generated that, much later, are induced to undergo mitosis again and, in due course, produce a multipolar mitosis. This might take place under the influence of a local stimulus such as trauma or inflammation or of a general change in the body such as puberty or pregnancy.

It seems to me that the malignant tumours that arise in skin naevi are of great interest in this respect. Hansemann claims that they do not develop in all kinds of naevi but only in those that contain peculiarly large cells. According to Hansemann, it is the presence of these cells that constitutes the risk of tumour formation. Is it not probable that these unusually large cells are tetraploids whose next division has to be a tetrapolar mitosis?

44. At first sight this proposal seems to be at loggerheads with the view adopted by Boveri in his introduction to this essay, namely that cells can go on multiplying for long periods, if not indefinitely, without specific stimulation (the work of Woodruff). The impulse to multiply is there regarded as an inherent property of the cells. But since the two 'stimuli' discussed here both produce derangements of cell division – the first an inhibition of cytoplasmic partitioning and the second an abnormal mitosis – it is not difficult to see how the two proposals can be reconciled.

13. The other observation that I have discussed above – that malignant tumours arise especially often at sites of chronic irritation – is readily understood in terms of our hypothesis after what has just been said about transient traumas. In the first place, chronic injury and the disturbances that it causes induce concomitant regeneration and a great deal of cell multiplication, which obviously presupposes cell division and the occurrence of abnormal divisions [45]. In the second place, the noxious influence itself will at the same time greatly facilitate the production of abnormal mitoses. We have already heard about squeezing, vigorous shaking and abnormal temperatures as agents that can give rise to multipolar mitoses in *Echinus* embryos, but we must here draw attention to the important finding that we owe above all to the investigations of the Hertwig brothers (Hertwig and Hertwig, 1887), namely that other poisons such as quinine, chloral hydrate, morphine, nicotine and no doubt many others have the same effect. Recently, O. and G. Hertwig (Hertwig, 1910, 1911, 1912) produced multipolar mitoses in sea urchin eggs by using radium to irradiate the sperm before fertilisation. I have myself confirmed that radium can enhance the production of tetrapolar mitoses in fertilised *Ascaris* eggs.

If one compares these agents with chronic irritants that, as is well known, often give rise to cancer, then the correspondence is striking. Carcinoma of the gall bladder in tightly corseted women, especially when combined with gallstones, might illustrate the effect of squeezing. Laceration might well have the same effect, for we learn that in India it is only at the root of the right-hand horn by which the cattle are tethered that skin carcinomas arise. Raised temperature seems to produce carcinoma of the œsophagus in Chinese men who eat their rice as hot as possible, whereas

45. Boveri had no doubt that cell multiplication in humans took place only by means of binary fission, discovered by Robert Remak in the middle of the nineteenth century. [For a referenced account of the work of Remak, see Harris, H. (1999) *The Birth of the Cell*, Yale University Press.] But the text here still leaves open the possibility, albeit an extremely unlikely one, that other modes of cell multiplication might exist. Perhaps there were still vocal doubters in the medical community in 1914.

the women let it cool first [46]. Cancers resulting from radiation need no more than a mention. The connection between cancer and certain chemical irritants is even clearer than it is between cancer and the physical agents I have mentioned. I need only refer to the cancers of paraffin workers.

As I have mentioned above, in all these cases, the malignant tumour never seems to be the direct consequence of the irritant; this itself merely produces inflammatory and ulcerative reactions and concomitant abundant cell division. It is my view that the specific damage then operates on these dividing cells, usually by suppressing the process of cell division itself. And the resulting tetraploid cells are driven to divide by the continuous proliferation provoked by the recurrent irritation. This opens the door for the production of sarcomatous or carcinomatous progenitor cells.

But I do not want to exclude the other possibility, that the abnormal stimulus might induce simultaneous multiple division of the centrosomes, which would lead to abnormal chromosome combinations even more easily [47].

Apart from the variety of the tumours that originate in the one tissue, their frequent occurrence against a background of chronic irritation is the characteristic that supports our hypothesis most strongly.

14. Parasites of all sorts, from bacteria, moulds and protozoa to worms and arthropods, have been touted as causes of malignant tumours. Most of these claims have been rejected. It does, however, appear to be the case that *Distomum haematobium* [48] can cause

---

46. Given the anecdotal state of medical epidemiology at the time, these crude correlations are not more primitive than the epidemiological 'breakthroughs' that pepper our present daily newspapers.

47. It is not surprising that Boveri draws attention to the possibility that the centrosome might be involved in generating malignancy. It was Boveri's own work, published at the turn of the century, that clarified the role of this organelle in cell division [Boveri, T. (1901) *Naturwissenschaften* 35, 1]. However, perhaps because no experimental evidence supported the idea that centrosome abnormalities might lead to cancer, this suggestion met little response for more than half a century. It has nonetheless been resurrected in recent years as a concomitant of the renewed interest in aneuploidy.

carcinomas and sarcomas, and some nematodes also appear to do so. As far as the latter are concerned, the systematic experiments of Fibiger [49] have recently shown that a species of *Spiroptera* that parasitises the fundus of the stomach can cause, among other pathological changes, metastatic carcinomas. Fibiger himself is convinced that the parasites exert their effect by means of a poison that they produce, and he classifies this mode of action as a form of chronic irritation. I regard it as highly probable that this interpretation holds for all cases where parasites are thought to be the cause of tumours. A carcinoma produced by parasites is in the same category as a paraffin-worker's cancer or a pipe-smoker's cancer.

Even though, from our point of view, these connections do not appear to need deep analysis, Fibiger's description of his findings does require further discussion. In the rat stomach, the *Spiroptera* produces an inflammatory reaction and gives rise to papillomas, often very large ones. Fibiger regards this papillomatosis as a preliminary stage in the development of malignant newgrowths. If this statement is true, then it ruins our hypothesis. For that would mean that the carcinoma is an exacerbation of a pre-existing malady that becomes apparent in the papillomas. But, in my opinion, the carcinoma is as fundamentally different from the papilloma as it is from the flat epithelium of the ventricular fundus. The inflammation and proliferation produced by the parasites simply provide the best possible preconditions for the generation of strictly localised carcinomas. As in all the other cases in which a carcinoma arises against a background of inflammation or from within a benign tumour, our hypothesis assumes that it has a completely localised origin in one cell with a specific abnormal chromosome constitution.

---

48. This is a trematode flatworm with two suckers.

49. Johannes Fibiger's first paper on the alleged stomach cancers produced in rats by a species of *Spiroptera* appeared in 1913, one year before Boveri's monograph. Fibiger's publications created a sensation at the time; although Boveri could hardly ignore them, he nonetheless treats the discovery with some reserve. In due course, Fibiger's claims were comprehensively demolished, but that did not prevent him being awarded the Nobel Prize in Physiology or Medicine in 1926.

It therefore seems to me that Fibiger's discoveries do not contradict the interpretation I have given. His findings, as far as I can see, do not support the idea that the carcinomatous process is an exacerbation of the papillomatous process. Indeed, Fibiger expressly emphasised that, in cases where carcinoma is undoubtedly present, other changes in the stomach are not so striking as they are in cases of simple papillomatosis. So, for the time being, it is right to assume that, in one or a few sites, the rapid proliferation of the epithelium gives rise to abnormal mitoses and hence to carcinomatous progenitor cells. It is the proliferation of these cells that is responsible for the whole cancerous disease.

It is especially interesting that Fibiger finds that the metastases derived from the stomach carcinoma are free from parasites. It could not be clearer that the parasite is merely an indirect cause that might eventually lead to the production of malignant cells. Once these are formed, they proliferate without the need for any external stimulus, entirely as a consequence of their own inherent properties.

15. If what I have said about parasites is correct then the question of contagiousness can easily be brought into line with our hypothesis. If any parasite has the power to induce the formation of malignant tumours, whether this is due to the provision of a stimulus that suppresses cell division, or one that induces abnormal multiple division of the centrosomes, or one that causes the degeneration of certain chromosomes, then the transmission of that parasite to another individual exposes that individual to the same peril. The facts we have at present do not seem to me to support anything more than this kind of indirect contagion.

16. In our view, tumours that arise as a sequel to other tumours are explicable in the same way as tumours that arise due to parasites. We have already discussed how, according to our chromosome hypothesis, the cells of malignant tumours release abnormal products that differ from one tumour to another and hence produce different effects on their surroundings. In certain cases, these effects must be classed as a form of chronic irritation just like noxious substances introduced into the tissues from the

outside. We have already tried to explain how the latter lead to the formation of tumours.

Bashford has found that there are strains of carcinoma in the mouse that, albeit very rarely and after a certain delay, rapidly give rise to sarcomas each time they are transplanted into a new host. The precise timing of the transition to sarcoma might raise doubts about our interpretation of events. A decision about this matter can only be made if we have a detailed understanding of what goes on. If it should turn out that all the sarcomas produced from the one carcinoma are of the same kind, this, coupled with the apparent consistency with which the sarcomas appear on transplantation, would indicate that the sarcomas arise in a more direct way than by selection out of a large number of random chromosome aberrations. And here perhaps the interpretation that we proposed for the occurrence of multiple and diffuse tumours might again be applicable. There, we learned that a cytoplasmic factor that we could not exactly specify acts on different chromosomes in different ways so that at mitosis some pass to the two daughter cells in the usual manner whereas others pass undivided to one or other daughter cell depending on where they happen to be. Is it not conceivable that the metabolic products released from certain mouse carcinomas might so alter the cytoplasm of neighbouring connective tissue cells that certain chromosomes might default in the way they do in sea urchin eggs? If we accept this point of view, then the production of cells with specific chromosomal defects would be such a tremendously frequent occurrence that, so long as one of these specific defects is what is required to generate a sarcoma, then after a certain time a tumour of this sort, or indeed several, would be expected in every case.

But we cannot categorically reject the other possibility, namely that a stimulus emanating from the carcinoma might elicit such rapid cell multiplication and at the same time so many abnormal cell divisions that the chromosome combinations that determine sarcomas would in all probability occur often enough to explain the phenomenon described by Bashford. Bashford states that an adenocarcinoma that he has studied has, over the years, produced spindle-cell, round-cell and pleomorphic-cell sarcomas. According to our hypothesis, this would mean that the progenitor cells of these sarcomas had received different combinations of chromosomes. This would perhaps support the second of our two possibilities, although it does not completely exclude the first.

17. The incidence of malignant tumours in different tissues is highly variable, and it seems to me in the light of our foregoing observations that this variation in the susceptibility of different tissues to tumour formation runs parallel, on the whole, to the frequency with which cell division takes place within them. In tissues where cells almost never divide, malignant tumours are very rare; they become more frequent if the tissue is forced to increase the rate of cell division to replace dead cells. If chronic irritation stimulates cell division in such tissues even further, then the probability that malignant tumours will occur rises still more. But the best soil for the growth of malignant tumours seems to be when the chronic irritation that leads to cell proliferation at the same time harbours a factor that has the power to produce abnormalities in the process of mitosis. Given what I have already said, it is remarkable how good the correlation is between this sequence of events and our hypothesis.

18. Despite this not-negligible regularity, there is something about the occurrence of malignant tumours that is much more striking, something that you might call capriciousness. We have already alluded to this in passing, but it merits a more coherent review.

Malignant tumours, especially carcinomas, are notably a disease of old age; but they also occur with all their characteristic features in young individuals, even in embryos. Indeed, they appear to be even more devastating in the young. They are found especially frequently at sites of chronic irritation. However, in many places where this has gone on for a long time, they do not arise; and, *vice versa*, they can appear in places where chronic irritation has certainly never taken place. Malignant tumours are often found in circumstances that make one think that they may have arisen from arrested embryonic cells [50], but in most cases a connection of this sort can be excluded. And if it is indeed the case that we can no longer doubt that malignant proliferation of tissues can be produced by parasites, a parasitic origin seems nonetheless to be inadmissible for the great majority of malignant tumours.

So it is not surprising if the most scrupulous authorities declare that a unitary cause for malignant tumours or, to narrow the range, a unitary cause for carcinomas, cannot be accepted[51]. But, in my view, this statement can only be right if one ignores the final, immediate cause. For if malignant tumours or, once again, carcinomas in particular, despite their variety represent a cellular aberration of the one kind, and not some sort of unnatural grouping of different maladies, then these tumours must have an immediate cause in common. Embryonic deviation or ageing of tissues, transient injury and chronic irritation, and whatever else can reasonably count as a causative factor in the development of malignant newgrowths, must produce the same aberrations in the cells if the consequences really are the same. As Borst puts it: 'The causes may be very varied and may lack a specific character – but the nature of the cellular aberration is certainly specific.'

That highly variable influences can in fact produce essentially the same effect is shown by an example that at this point is all the more apt as it bears on the matter around which everything in this essay turns – the inappropriately constituted chromosome complex. Double fertilisation of a sea urchin egg generally leads to the formation of a pathological product that perishes after a few days. An identical effect is often produced if, during its first division, a normally fertilised sea urchin egg is vigorously shaken. What could appear more different than the penetration of two spermatozoa into one egg and the effect of shaking a fertilised egg in the

50. There was once great enthusiasm for the theory that cancers arose from embryonic remnants ('embryonale Reste'). Boveri does not share this enthusiasm, but admits the possibility. The recent resurgence of interest in pluripotent stem cells prompts the observation that, if 'embryonic remnants' are viewed as entities that retain embryonic characteristics, the distinction between pluripotent stem cells and embryonic remnants appears less categorical.

51. This clinical platitude is still advanced from time to time with all the gravity of a deep insight. It would be astonishing, would it not, if different cancers in different places produced the same symptomatology?

process of dividing into two? But these two fundamentally different events nonetheless have essentially the same result: they both give rise to a tetrapolar mitosis and in this way produce an abnormal chromosome constitution in the daughter cells. The same aberration in both cases is without doubt the cause of the same disease in both cases.

Our hypothesis stipulates that the genesis of a malignant tumour requires a specific wrongly constituted chromosome complex and, as we have shown above, one that can be produced not only in different ways, but whose origin is largely a matter of chance. So it is altogether appropriate to call that event 'capricious' as we did earlier.

For, if my assumption is correct, the legacy that a tumour acquires is more or less comparable with the blind withdrawal of a particular number from a sack containing a thousand. One might try to do this hundreds of times and never select the right number, yet someone else might try only once and get it first time. In fact, the element of lottery pertains to the origin of malignant tumours in a number of ways. The very possibility that multipolar mitoses might arise, insofar as they are produced by the inhibition of cell division, is determined in large measure by chance, as it depends on whether the insult is severe enough during the brief period in which the cell is being partitioned. If a tetraploid cell is formed as a result of this insult, it will nonetheless be a matter of chance whether this particular cell receives a stimulus that induces it to divide. And if it gets that far, then the real game of dice begins in the multipolar mitosis, for then the outcome depends on whether a combination of chromosomes happens to come together in such a way in one of the daughter cells that it generates the properties characteristic of malignancy. The more abnormal cell divisions there are in a tissue, the greater the probability will of course be that the required combination will turn up; but it is conceivable that, despite the continuous iteration of abnormal mitoses, it might never do so. By contrast, a single multipolar mitosis taking place in healthy tissue, perhaps the result of simultaneous multiple division of the centrosome, could give rise to the cell that originates the malignant tumour.

Whether our hypothesis is right or wrong, I am convinced that any theory of tumour formation will have to accommodate a step that has the character of a lottery.

19. The fact to which I referred earlier, namely that the incidence of sarcomas and carcinomas, but especially the latter, increases with age, is so striking that if our assumption cannot also account for this phenomenon, then we must ask whether this phenomenon is at least consistent with it. Here, the most important consideration for us is that, although malignant tumours do arise more easily in ageing individuals, they grow more rapidly in young ones, as experiments with grafts[52] have shown us. This contrast, it seems to me, points to a relationship between the origin of malignant tumours and their subsequent behaviour that is entirely consistent with our hypothesis. The finding that age produces more favourable conditions for the generation of malignant tumours readily becomes comprehensible if one considers what happens in analogous experiments with egg cells. Just as there are ageing tissue cells, so there are also ageing eggs. After the centriole has been organised, the longer an egg cell has to wait for the arrival of the spermatozoon, the weaker its resistance will be to its eventual disintegration. An ageing egg of this sort can offer no resistance to the calamitous entry of several spermatozoa, and it is much more susceptible to noxious influences than a young cell. My experiments indicate that the inhibition of cytoplasmic partitioning by appropriate procedures, and hence the production of a situation that leads to a tetraploid mitosis at the next cell division, is more easily accomplished in an aged egg than in a young one. If we can assume that much the same thing holds true for ageing tissue cells, and it certainly looks like it, then that might be enough to explain the greater frequency of malignant tumours in old age.

20. A final argument that I believe I can regard as a support for my assumption is the outcome of observations on chromosome

52. It is not clear what grafting experiments Boveri is referring to, and he gives no reference. The concept of histoincompatibility had not yet appeared over the horizon, and it is doubtful whether any grafting experiments at that time would have had much probative value. Perhaps he is referring to the vegetative propagation of plants, but, if so, it is not easy to see a relevance to the cancer problem.

number and nuclear size in carcinomas. Long ago, Hansemann drew attention to the fact that mitoses with raised or reduced chromosome numbers are to be found in malignant tumours. Borst, too, states that one often observes an easily detectable increase in chromosome number in proliferating tissues, and less often a reduced chromosome number. Although these findings still need elaboration, even in their crude form they do offer strong support for our hypothesis. And the same can be said for the recent measurements of the size of the nuclei in carcinomas. I was able to show (1889, 1902) that in sea urchin eggs, *ceteris paribus*, the size of the nuclei was proportional to the number of chromosomes that they contained. Thus, owing to the very frequent unequal allocation of the chromosomes to the primary blastomeres, a larva formed from a dispermic egg may be composed of three or four regions with nuclei (and cells) of different sizes. That this proportionality holds for vertebrates has since been shown by Brachet and Herlant and by G. Hertwig. It is certainly probable that, in man too, and not only in immature tissues but also in mature ones, the size of the nuclei is similarly dependent on the number of chromosomes. In considering this question, the observations on nuclear size in tumour cells are of great significance in terms of our hypothesis. After Heiberg had found that the nuclei of cancer cells were generally larger than those of the tissue from which the cancer arose, Borst induced his pupil Nomikos to carry out measurements on a very extensive range of material. It turned out, in confirmation of Heiberg's results, that the nuclei of many carcinomas are larger than those of the tissues from which they were derived, and usually larger than the nuclei of benign epitheliomas. In many carcinomas, however, the nuclei are of normal size and, rarely, they are even smaller than the nuclei of the tissue of origin.

For the cancer researcher seeking a comprehensive morphological feature to characterise tumour cells, this finding, like so many previous ones, must come once again as a disappointment. But, if we look at tumours from the point of view of our hypothesis and accept the proposition that the proportionality between nuclear size and chromosome number holds true for grown men [53], then these results are exactly what you would expect. Our hypothesis, admittedly, does not permit us to decide *a priori* what nuclear sizes (and chromosome numbers) are most likely to be found in carcinomas. And we must remember that in an abnormally constituted nucleus the normal ratio of nuclear size to chromosome number might not hold. But there is one postulate that we cannot avoid: nuclei of different sizes are present in different malignant tumours. We know from experiments on merogony and artificial parthenogenesis that a cell with a haploid nucleus, which is one containing half the chromosome number found in tissue cells, can be normal. One can hardly assume that this would not apply to the tissue cells of man. Since, in my view, a malignant tissue cell is one in which at least one chromosome is missing, it must in theory be possible that there are tumours whose nuclei are less than half as big as those of the normal tissue from which the tumour is derived*. However, one must bear in mind that if, on the one hand, certain chromosomes must be missing in a tumour cell then, on the other hand, others must be present if the cell is to remain viable. Since the composition of the chromosome complex that multipolar mitosis allocates to each of the daughter cells is essentially fortuitous, it is obvious that the daughter cell that receives the largest number of chromosomes has the best chance of survival. And that might explain why the nuclei in the majority of carcinomas are larger than those in the tissue of origin. But, as I have explained, the combination required to produce a tumour may be assembled with far fewer chromosomes, so one can understand why carcinomas with smaller nuclei than normal, although uncommon, are sometimes found.

---

*What the ratio between haploid and diploid nuclei might be has to be determined for each case. In sea urchin larvae, it is the surface area of the nucleus that is proportional to the chromosome number; in other cases it is the nuclear volume.

53. The German text has 'erwachsenden Menschen' which would mean 'growing men'. But in the light of the preceding paragraph this does not make sense. My guess is that this is a misprint for 'erwachsenen Menschen', which means 'grown men' and makes more sense.

V. Consideration
of some objections

It is not my intention to offer a preconceived opposition to any objection that clinicians or pathologists might make to my hypothesis. I merely wish to discuss certain misgivings that are supported by cytological observations and that, in my opinion, are responsible for the fact that the explanation attempted in this essay was, from the very beginning, judged to be unacceptable.

The first objection, which I have received many times by word of mouth, is that atypical mitoses are in no way specific to malignant tumours. Such mitoses can also be found in benign proliferations or inflammatory conditions or even in completely normal tissues; by contrast, they are not always seen in malignant tumours. I myself can confirm the last of these observations. When, 26 years ago, while I was busy studying the composition of multipolar mitotic figures, I came across reports of abnormalities of this sort in carcinomas, I cut sections of several fresh specimens of carcinoma removed at operation that were put at my disposal in Nussbaum's clinic in Munich. I was unable to find a single multipolar or asymmetrical mitosis in any of these specimens.

I would like to think that the explanations given in the previous chapter will have already made it clear to the reader that, according to my hypothesis, atypical mitoses are by no means to be regarded as an essential property of malignant tumours. Indeed, the opposite is the case, a matter that I propose to discuss presently. Moreover, the occurrence of abnormal mitoses of this sort in otherwise healthy or diseased tissues constitutes one of the most important pieces of evidence in support of my hypothesis. For my hypothesis claims no more than that a multipolar or asymmetrical mitosis in any hitherto normal cell might lead to the formation of a malignant tumour, but not at all that it must do so. If then malignant tumours arise preferentially at sites of inflammation, if benign proliferations suddenly become malignant, or if, finally, a carcinoma or a sarcoma arises in normal tissue in which there has been no previous disease, then it is precisely the presence of abnormal mitoses in completely or at least relatively normal tissues that, according to my hypothesis, must be regarded as the origin of the malignant tumours.

Here there might be a second objection: that atypical mitoses occur much too often for them to be accepted as the cause of malignant tumours. Against this view, however, one must point out that analogous experiments on sea urchin eggs, as well as general considerations, lead to the well-founded conclusion that abnormal nuclear divisions do not, in most cases, produce the combination of chromosomes that is required to generate a malignant cell. Many of the cells formed by multipolar mitoses may have been allocated an assembly of chromosomes that produces a nearly normal cell, but much more often a cell that is no longer viable. Nothing argues against the supposition that on average only one in a thousand or even a hundred thousand abnormal mitoses generates the chromosome combination that keeps a cell alive and at the same time makes it abnormal in a quite specific way. That is why I regard the numerous observations of atypical cell divisions in non-malignant tissues not as an objection to my hypothesis but as an important argument in its favour.

To demonstrate the irrelevance of multipolar mitoses to the tumour problem, attention has been drawn in many quarters to the situation in leucocytes where some people have imagined that this form of mitosis is the normal mode of multiplication of these cells. But here the important investigations of M. Heidenhain (Heidenhain, 1894) have to be taken into account. Heidenhain showed that the multipolar mitoses produced in leucocytes[54] by inhibition of cell partitioning give rise to giant cells containing several sets of a completely normal chromosome complement[55]. Such cells, according to my hypothesis, would, of course, remain

54. It is of interest that Boveri does not distinguish between one kind of leucocyte and another. Paul Ehrlich had already established the individual character of lymphocytes and of neutrophil, basophil and eosinophil granulocytes as early as the 1870s. But the identification of blood-borne monocytes and their connection to tissue macrophages was not made until much later. Neutrophil granulocytes, by far the commonest leucocytes in the blood, do not multiply at all and do not give rise to multinucleate cells.

healthy unless they are impaired for some other reason. If, however, the multipolar mitosis in a leucocyte is followed by a simultaneous multiple division of the cytoplasm, who would wish to assert that the daughter cells would function normally? Perhaps they might even survive only for so long as they retain a supply of substances left over in their cytoplasm by the chromosomes that are now missing. But it seems to me that one cannot exclude the possibility that the simultaneous multiple divisions of the leucocytes might once in a way give rise to cells that are viable, but altered in their properties, in particular cells with a propensity for unrestrained multiplication. Indeed, leukaemias have been regarded as malignant newgrowths of leucocytes.

As for the frequent occurrence of atypical mitoses in tumours, however, my view is that this is not at all an existential characteristic of the tumour, but merely a symptom of a certain diseased state in the tumour cells. It is a symptom that perhaps leads one to suppose that a tendency to divide abnormally was already present in the cells of the tissue of origin and that it was this that generated the cell that gave rise to the tumour. But the actual growth of the tumour can, according to my hypothesis, proceed only by regular bipolar mitosis. The multipolar or asymmetrical mitoses in tumour cells might, however, occasionally convert the original phenotype of the tumour into a new one, presumably always a less differentiated one. In general though, it can be assumed that the chromosome complexes produced by new assortments of a chromatin constitution that is already defective would no longer leave the cells viable. And here we come to a point that seems to me of particular importance. Emphasis is laid on three properties that are thought to be characteristic of most tumours: the frequent occurrence of atypical mitoses; the great structural variability of the individual tumour cells, which is especially obvious in the spread of nuclear sizes; and the widespread evidence of degeneration. I like to think that these phenomena are causally related in

55. The mitosis in leucocytes described by Heidenhain must have taken place in macrophages, and it is these cells that form multinucleate 'giants'. For decades there was argument about whether these giants were formed by fusion of mononuclear cells or by nuclear division unaccompanied by cytoplasmic partitioning.

that they are ramifications of one and the same process. The variable distribution of chromosomes produced by the abnormal mitoses that occur in cancer cells gives rise to cells with an extreme range of nuclear sizes, cells that at the same time lose the original morphological characteristics of the tumour cells and replace them with others, and usually cells with very limited viability.

To put it briefly, the cells derived from a tumour cell by multipolar mitosis are in the vast majority of cases no longer tumour cells; paradoxical as it may sound, atypical mitosis that in normal tissue can give rise to this calamitous abnormality can only be regarded as a therapeutic factor in a tumour that has already been established. In fact, one can imagine that if in a malignant tumour multipolar mitoses were the rule, the tumour would gradually undergo involution of its own accord, and if the products of its decomposition were removed quickly enough, a cure might be achieved.

X-rays and radium radiation are said to have both the power to produce cancer and also the power to heal it. This curiously ambivalent effect might be explicable in part by the ability of these rays to produce abnormal mitoses. Under their influence, normal cells give rise to malignant cells, but malignant cells give rise to cells that are no longer viable. Of course, the unusually rapid cure produced by radioactive substances can only be mediated by a direct effect of the rays on resting tumour cells.

৵৵৵

No doubt the most important cytological objection to my hypothesis stems from the various authoritative opinions in pathological anatomy concerning amitotic division. If the resting nucleus is ubiquitously constructed in the manner that the theory of chromosome individuality presupposes, then the simple direct partitioning of the nucleus, with the corresponding partitioning of the cytoplasm that it entails, must give rise to daughter cells whose chromosome constitution will in general deviate from the norm in the same way as the daughter cells produced by multipolar mitosis. For, depending on the fortuitous bilateral position of the chromosomes in the resting nucleus and on the direction of the partitioning, the two daughter cells will necessarily receive very different chromosome complements. And if, as follows from our hypothesis, the individual chromosomes have different properties and manage to function normally only when present in specific combinations, then, in general, the cells produced by direct partitioning of the nucleus must be pathological and doomed to die.

Now what do we really know about amitotic division and its consequences [56]? As far as I am aware there has been only a single description of the chromosomal consequences of an undoubtedly direct partitioning of the nucleus and that is the observation made recently in the Zoological Institute at Würzburg by G. Kautzsch (Kautzsch, 1912). This study centres on the division of the abnormally large centrioles seen in the developing eggs of *Ascaris megalocephala*. Because they have an ample amount of cytoplasm, these abortive eggs do manage to initiate some parthenogenetic development, albeit of an extremely rudimentary sort. The two chromosomes associated with the huge centriole then prepare to undergo mitotic division and indeed do split into two daughter chromosomes, so that there are now four. But the separation of the chromatids does not take place because the achromatic elements of the mitotic apparatus are missing, and all four daughter chromosomes are then reunited in a single resting nucleus.

Frequently, soon after the nucleus is formed, the cytoplasm is partitioned into two separate pieces and, if the furrow passes through the nucleus, it divides this too into two more or less unequal parts. In this way, amitosis produces two nucleated daughter cells. Each of these daughter nuclei then undergoes a mitotic division once again, which has the important consequence that each nucleus now no longer contains the characteristic two or four chromosomes of *Ascaris* cells, but any assortment

56. Although Hofmeister had described and illustrated mitotic figures in plant cells as early as 1848 [Hofmeister, W. (1848) *Bot. Zeit.* 6, cols 423, 649, 670], and Flemming had finally delineated all the stages of mitosis ('indirect' division of the nucleus) by 1879 [Flemming, W. (1879) *Arch. f. mikr. Anat.* 16, 302] and had argued strongly that this was the only way in which plant and animal cells divided, it seems that in the backwaters of pathological anatomy there were still voices in 1914 that argued in favour of 'direct' partitioning of the nucleus. It is obvious that Boveri will have none of it and accepts as fact only a bizarre situation in abortive Ascaris eggs.

of chromosomes so long as the total number in both cells adds up to four (i.e. the number that the nucleus had before it was 'directly' partitioned). Even more telling is the fact that when the two nuclei formed by 'direct' partitioning prepare for mitosis, one of the chromosomes often sustains a fracture, and the segment broken off may pass to one daughter cell and the rest of the chromosome to the other. You could not find a better piece of evidence to illustrate the validity of the idea that in the impenetrable resting nucleus there are a number of independent regions, each of which emanates from a chromosome visible in the preceding mitosis and each of which condenses into the same chromosome at the next mitosis.

What nuclei containing a defective chromatin constitution of this sort can achieve cannot regrettably be established in this case as the embryos stop developing very early for other reasons.

If we now turn to the 'direct' cell division that is supposed to be a normal process in metazoa, one must ask whether or not we are dealing with a course of events such as I have just described. Child (Child, 1907) claims that in the tapeworm *Moniezia* mitotic and amitotic divisions can alternate in an arbitrary fashion but that in all mitotic divisions the characteristic chromosome number for that species reappears. (Child has endeavoured to generalise his results as far as possible.) Much the same sort of thing is said by Shearer to occur during egg formation in the worm *Dinophilus*.

If this is so, then the 'direct' division that in these two cases is intercalated between two mitotic divisions must be a different process from that described in all its stages by Kautzsch. Since the latter case has made it clear that 'direct' division of a normal resting nucleus transmits to the two daughter cells nuclei that are reduced to partial nuclei, each being the complement of the other, something very special must have happened in a resting nucleus in which 'direct' partitioning transmits a complete chromosome set to each of the daughter cells. One could imagine that the individual chromosomes vaporise, so to speak, into tiny particles and that these particles then form an intimate amalgam. If this amalgam were split into two halves by any transverse cross-section, each half would receive approximately the same number of particles from every chromosome and, if the particles then come together again in appropriate combinations, the end result would be much the same as that produced by mitotic division.

It is clear that 'direct' division of this kind would not affect our tumour hypothesis. If, on the other hand, it can be shown that mammalian daughter cells produced in the manner described by Kautzsch remain alive and are in other ways normal, then our hypothesis must be wrong.

We must therefore consider how we should assess the numerous reports of 'direct' division in mammalian tissues. But first we must cast a glance at the above-mentioned observations of Child on the sex organs of *Moniezia* because these provide much more favourable material than mammalian tissue for the precise delineation of the whole course of events. Nonetheless, and despite the fact that Child's observations give the impression of having been made with great care, no actual proof of 'direct' division is given. To provide proof, as I have pointed out elsewhere, one must demonstrate: that the binucleate condition is really the result of 'direct' division; that an area of cytoplasm is delimited around each of these nuclei; and that the cells formed then undergo mitotic division and thereby have the normal chromosome number. Child has not managed to provide any of these indispensable pieces of evidence.

It is in the nature of things that the claims concerning 'direct' cell division in mammals are no better off. I have the impression that most of these authors were convinced that 'direct' division had already been demonstrated beyond doubt by their predecessors and they have therefore made do with inadequate evidence. I must stress once again that lobulated nuclei or binucleate cells, and the most beautiful series of pictures arranged to show the transformation of a single nucleus into two nuclei, cannot in themselves provide a shred of evidence for 'direct' division even of the nucleus [57]. Depending on the bilateral disposition of the chromosomes allocated to a daughter cell by mitosis, all sorts of nuclei can

57. The besetting sin of traditional histopathology – to infer what has taken place in a tissue from the examination of static stained sections.

be formed showing varying degrees of constriction; and, if the daughter chromosomes happen to find themselves in two outlying groups, two nuclei may be formed that do not fuse during the whole of the cellular resting phase. But even where a resting nucleus really has been cut into two by 'direct' partitioning, the main question remains unanswered. The nucleus of a metazoan cell is not an organ that ensures cell division, as is the case in some protozoa; two nuclei in a metazoan cell do not at all presage partitioning of the cytoplasm that lies between them. In any case, in all the instances that I have myself been able to follow in detail, no change occurs in the further development of binucleate metazoan cells (in *Ascaris* and *Triton*) until the next mitosis when both nuclei disaggregate and all the chromosomes are drawn into a simple bipolar mitotic figure.

Therefore, to demonstrate 'direct' division, you absolutely have to demonstrate partitioning of the cell between the two nuclei. Even so, there is still the possibility of error. By the time the cytoplasm undergoes partitioning, daughter cells produced by mitotic division might again have passed far enough into the resting phase that it is impossible to decide whether the nuclei were formed mitotically or amitotically. Indeed, even if a connection persists between two resting nuclei and there is partitioning or contraction of the cytoplasm between them, this does not prove that 'direct' division has occurred. Long ago I showed that, during the segmentation of the egg in *Ascaris*, such appearances may follow a mitosis if in one or more chromosomes the process of splitting is delayed. This has since been demonstrated in other material.

A mammalian tissue with which I have myself experimented is the corneal epithelium of the rabbit. In a recent study of regeneration in this epithelium, Juselius (Juselius, 1910) has claimed that to begin with mitoses do occur, but these soon peter out and replacement of the cells that have been removed then takes place essentially by means of 'direct' division. There is not a shred of evidence in Juselius's paper to support this contention. One gets the impression that he attributes the major role in the regenerative process to amitosis because he sees so few mitoses. But in this he is mistaken. I have repeated these experiments as he described them but with one modification. I examined the cornea not in histological sections but in flat preparations of the epithelium. If the connective tissue elements of the cornea are removed as far as possible and the staining is not too dark, then with good illumination the flattened sheet can be analysed in detail, and the number and distribution of the mitoses can be determined much more easily and much more accurately than can be achieved by reconstruction of a long series of sections. These flat preparations then show that for at least seven days there is vigorous mitotic activity in the vicinity of the defect and no evidence at all of amitotic activity. I can therefore no longer doubt that the cell multiplication set going to replace the missing epithelial cells takes place exclusively by mitosis*.

* I should like to take this opportunity to communicate briefly a finding of mine that has not yet been published. I began my investigations on mammalian epithelium with the lens epithelium of the rabbit. One of my colleagues, C. von Hess, kindly showed me how, if you let out the vitreous fluid and rub the cocainised cornea with a blunted glass rod, you can produce ragged defects in the lens epithelium. Regeneration by means of mitotic division of healthy cells begins at the edges of the defects and moves in a very regular fashion towards the periphery. Depending on how much time has gone by, this process produces parallel bands of mitoses in the neighbourhood of the defect, but at an ever-increasing distance from its edge. These bands are sometimes astonishingly regular, but more often blurred. I could not resist giving this phenomenon the name 'karyokinetic wave'. Although the first wave arises at the edge of the defect, the second or third waves are less distinct. I happened to mention this finding to my colleague Professor Borst and it was he who drew my attention to the above-mentioned work of Juselius, who had described something similar in the epithelium of the cornea. Indeed, I found that he had described much the same sort of thing as a 'karyokinetic wave', but he thought it moved in the opposite direction to what I had found in the lens epithelium. He claimed that a few hours after the operation, mitoses occur at the limbus and then move towards the edge of the defect, whereas those at the periphery peter out. My own observations on preparations fixed at the times indicated by Juselius did not provide me with the slightest evidence to support his claim, and I can only explain his results, apart from the unsuitability of histological sections for the investigation of this problem, by concluding that he has been deceived by fortuitous coincidences. Even in completely intact and undisturbed corneal epithelium there are always mitoses, probably most numerous in young animals. They are to be found all over, but are especially common at the periphery. I do not doubt that it was the presence of these mitoses that put Juselius's idea into his head. In corneal epithelium too, the mitotic reaction to the defect begins close to its edge and proceeds towards the periphery, although in this case the wave is not as distinct as that seen in lens epithelium[58].

'Direct' nuclear division without cell partitioning does not of course affect my hypothesis any more than multiple mitotic division without cytoplasmic partitioning, as I have already explained, for in these cases the cells contain complete sets of chromosomes. The reports of 'direct' nuclear division in the regeneration of striated muscle should perhaps be considered from this point of view. In this case too, the nuclei that are formed remain together in one integral matrix of cytoplasm. But it seems to me that the role that amitotic nuclear division might play in the regenerative restoration of functional muscle fibres has not been fully explained by Schminke's investigations.

In the end, we have to say pretty much what we said about abnormal mitoses in normal tissues: if 'direct' cell divisions really do take place in mammals in the manner described by Kautzsch, who knows what becomes of such cells? Who can say that they do not promptly perish? They might indeed still remain alive for a while, just as the blastomeres of dispermic sea urchin eggs do. These blastomeres, despite their defective chromatin constitution, manage to complete a normal cell division, but after repeated mitotic binary fission they suddenly sicken and die. It is altogether possible, as the survival of anucleate protozoal fragments have shown us, that the cytoplasm retains a supply of material emanating from the nucleus that was present at an earlier stage and that this material is not all used up until some time has elapsed.

In considering these matters, it would even be consistent with my view of the composition of the nucleus if 'direct' division actually had a physiological role, that is, if you made an exception for the production of cells like those of the epidermis of mammals, which have to die before they can fulfil their normal function. Only the deepest layer of the epidermis has to keep regenerating itself by means of cell divisions that yield daughter cells containing complete chromosome sets. But the cells that are programmed to migrate into the upper layers, and are thereby already doomed to an inexorable end, might still multiply for a while by a mech-

58. Although in Boveri's text this aside appears merely as a lengthy footnote, it remains the classical description of healing in an epithelial monolayer.

anism that generates only daughter cells that contain defective nuclei.

In summary, my conclusions are as follows:

- Amitotic nuclear division without subsequent cell division is of no consequence as far as our hypothesis is concerned.
- All claims relating to amitotic nuclear division followed by partitioning of the cytoplasm are to be treated with the utmost reserve. In so far as they deal with normal events, they are, in my view, for the most part rooted in error. But if this kind of division gives rise to impaired daughter cells, then that constitutes evidence in support of my theory.
- The 'direct' division of cells that for other reasons retain a limited potential for further survival could be entirely consistent with my ideas.
- The foregoing propositions refer to amitotic divisions that proceed in the manner described by Kautzsch in which the daughter cell receives only a fraction of the mother cell's chromosome complement. However, it is conceivable that a form of amitotic cell division might exist in which each of the daughter cells receives half of all the chromosome particles that the nucleus contains, even if the halving achieved is not as exact as that produced by mitosis. This course of events would not be in conflict with my hypothesis.

All in all, I am convinced that amitotic division does not pose any threat to the tumour hypothesis that I have presented.

VI. Conclusion

However incomplete these comments might still be, I hope they will be given credit for at least one thing: that they do not rely on some unique event, but endeavour to come to terms with a series of the most significant phenomena that characterise malignant tumours. Given the great variability of the facts that have to be explained, one would hardly expect *a priori* that a hypothesis of this kind would provide an immediate solution to every problem. This hypothesis would be worth exploring if it provided a coherent interpretation for several properties that had hitherto seemed unconnected and if it was at least compatible with the rest.

Regarding the latter qualification, my exposition could be extended in various directions. There is a great deal that I have not even touched upon: for example, tumour immunity or the mode of action of various medicaments. But, as far as I can see, there is for the time being not much more to be said other than that the tumour cells react in this way or that, and it seems to me that there is no fact that forces us to exclude the possibility that a particular pattern of behaviour might have its origin in our view of the special character of the nucleus. What is particularly interesting about the effect of radium and thorium on carcinomas is the observation of O. Hertwig and his collaborators, who showed that quite generally the deleterious effect of the irradiation acts primarily on the nucleus. It is not too far fetched to assume in the light of our hypothesis that the defective nucleus of the malignant tumour cell succumbs more easily to the impact of these rays than the nucleus of a normal cell. Here again the dispermic sea urchin eggs, which we have so often used for purposes of comparison in the course of our discussion, behave in much the same way. Even those few that manage to develop into something approaching normal plutei turn out to be more susceptible to detrimental influences than the products of monospermic eggs. The following observation struck me as particularly illuminating. In all the species that I have looked at, the dispermic eggs that divide into three produce a number of reasonably normal-looking larvae, even if their development is somewhat imperfect. According to our hypothesis, this means that in certain circumstances the tripolar mitosis produces three nuclei that do not of course contain an absolutely normal chromosome complex, but at least one that can sustain almost normal function as far as the pluteus stage. If one attempts to make an interspecific cross with dispermic eggs that divide into three, as I have often done, the embryos invariably perish, whereas monospermic interspecific crosses from the same parents invariably produce normal larvae. The only possible interpretation that can be given for this effect of interspecific crossing in these instances of dispermy is that the marginally abnormal chromosome constitution that can at a pinch fulfil its function in completely normal circumstances such as prevail in amphimixis within the one species, can no longer do so in the altered circumstances generated by the interspecific cross. And the damage done here by interspecific crossing might well be comparable with that done to malignant tumours by radioactive substances. The same might well be true for the specific effect that selenium has on certain mouse tumours, according to the experiments of A. von Wassermann. For here too, as Hansemann ascertained, it is in the nuclei of the tumour cells that the effect of selenium is first discernible.

What follows is a brief review of the sequence of ideas embodied in this essay.

We begin by assuming that the properties of malignant cells are due to an inherent defect. This defect is irreparable as is clear from the ultimate fate of these tumours, especially from their sequential transplantation from one individual to the next.

There is a great deal of evidence that irreparable cellular defects cannot be produced by injury to the cytoplasm alone. Yet, we know that we can produce defects in the nucleus that do not allow a return to normality. Chromosomes that are lost to the cell following abnormal mitosis cannot be reconstituted no matter how long these cells are propagated. And, for this reason, the nuclei generated by direct nuclear partitioning followed by cell division are actually partial nuclei in which not only missing chromosomes but also missing fragments of chromosomes cannot be replaced.

Such defects might have been regarded as of no consequence if, as we used to believe, all the chromosomes in a nucleus were essentially equivalent. However, we have compelling reasons for assuming that the individual chromosomes of metazoan nuclei have different properties. Their differences are not only quantitative, as appears to be the case in protozoa, but also qualitative. They are specialised in different ways and can only maintain the normality of the cell if they are present in a certain specific combination.

Experiments with sea urchin embryos have demonstrated that most chromosome combinations that deviate from the norm lead to the death of the cell, but there are some that allow the cell to survive but not to function normally. Among these are cases where the deviation from normality results in the dissolution of the tight apposition that characterises epithelial cells in normal development, a peculiarity that calls to mind the behaviour of certain malignant tumours. Admittedly, the principal characteristic of such tumours, namely unrestricted proliferation, could not be tested in sea urchin embryos.

Nuclear defects, such as I have described in sea urchins, are the result of multipolar mitoses. Since abnormalities of this sort are not infrequently found in malignant tumours, it is reasonable to suppose that there is some connection between them and the origin of tumours. The doubts that might be raised against this idea on cytological grounds I believe have been dealt with effectively in Chapter V.

But the essential element in our hypothesis is not the abnormal mitosis, but always a specific abnormal chromosome constitution. However this might arise, a particular tumour will be the result. Apart from multipolar mitosis, which might be produced either by simultaneous multiple division of the centrosome or by dislocation of the parallelism between division of the centrosome and that of the cell, it is primarily the asymmetrical mitoses that must be

75

reckoned with. Indeed, in a manner analogous to certain phenomena in sea urchins, these, being caused by a failure of specific chromosomes to divide properly, are much more likely to generate a tumour than the fortuitous division of the chromatin produced by multipolar mitoses. But the agencies that would have the most direct effect would be those that have the ability to destroy certain chromosomes within the cell, yet leave others unscathed.

For the time being, one cannot delineate our fundamental assumption more precisely. Like nuclear physiology, the pathology of the nucleus – which, in our view, is the area in which the theory of malignant tumours would fall – has hardly begun. Nonetheless, the assumption, in quite general terms, that there is a chromosomal defect, coupled with a description of how such defects can arise, does help us to understand many of the peculiarities of malignant tumours.

Above all, our hypothesis can explain the defective histological architecture and the altered biochemical properties of tumour cells. At the same time, it can account for the alterations that the tumour produces in its surrounding tissue.

The fact that there may be countless different abnormal chromosome combinations, of which the vast majority are, in our view, incompatible with the survival of the cell, provides us with a simple explanation for the varied nature of the malignant tumours that arise in the one tissue of origin.

There is a striking correspondence between experimental reagents that produce multipolar mitoses and the chronic irritants that have now been shown to have an undoubted role in the aetiology of malignant tumours.

On the other hand, the occasional appearance of an abnormal nuclear division in normal tissue provides a plausible explanation for the production of a malignant tumour at a site where an external causal factor is difficult to imagine. In any case, in the origin of malignant tumours, the factor that I previously described as 'capricious' fits our hypothesis extremely well.

There are also a number of other phenomena that can effortlessly be accommodated in our theory: for example, the generation of metastases, and the production of multiple and diffuse tumours as well as tumours made up of two or more cell types. Furthermore, the tumours produced by parasites or the emergence after transplantation of a tumour of a completely different kind might also be explicable in terms of our assumption.

The main thesis is admittedly hypothetical, namely whether an abnormal chromosome constitution can be produced such that the cells that harbour it are driven to unrestrained proliferation. This assumption must be made *ad hoc*, but there is much to be said for it. Above all, I regard it as beyond doubt that the tendency to multiply indefinitely is a primaeval property of cells and that the inhibition of multiplication in metazoan cells occurs secondarily under the influence of the environment [59]. Cells normally submit to this inhibition and reassert their original proliferative drive only when there are certain changes in their environment. If this is so, one must presuppose that there exists a specific cellular apparatus that is sensitive to conditions in the environment. Given such an apparatus, one must assume that it is susceptible to aberrations that incur the loss of sensitivity to the conditions of the environment. Then, the inherent proliferative drive of the cell is released and proceeds without taking any notice of the requirements of the rest of the body.

But to site this hypothetical regulatory apparatus in the cell nucleus seems to be justified by the fact that there are certainly connections between the chromatin and the regulation of cell division. So it is possible that specific changes in the constitution of the nucleus may produce the malfunction that results in the loss of reactivity to the state of the environment.

A question arises: is there some way to reach a firmer decision concerning the validity of the views I have put forward? In the light of all we know so far about malignant tumours, I do not see

59. Boveri ends as he began with a declaration of his fundamental view of cell multiplication – that to multiply is an inherent property of all cells, curbed in metazoa by the process of differentiation.

any possibility that we might be able to detect a malignant tumour *in statu nascendi* with the experimental methods currently available. In any case, this assertion is true if my hypothesis is correct. But, if there is no longer any doubt about the nature of proliferation, then the particular abnormal mitosis in which the tumour originates has long gone by. And even if one did have that mitosis before one's eyes, one would have no marker that might enable us to recognise it.

At best, there might be some hope of observing the genesis of a malignant tumour where an organ is transformed into a malignant tumour within a brief period and where the progenitor cells of the tumour are present in large numbers.

However, this apart, it is at least possible to submit my hypothesis to a more exacting examination than I have been able to do against the background of the facts known to me. There are, indeed, many ways of doing this. No doubt the most obvious is to enumerate the chromosomes with greater care and, where possible, with better methods than those available hitherto. I mentioned above that both abnormal chromosome numbers and abnormal nuclear dimensions are often found in tumours. With informative material it should be possible to make progress in this area. Nonetheless, for the time being, we will have to bear in mind what one might expect from studies of this kind. The finding that there is an approximately normal chromosome number in a malignant tumour, or indeed the occasional appearance of an exactly normal chromosome number, is not incompatible with our hypothesis. In a tetrapolar mitosis produced by suppression of cell division, the chromosomes might be distributed to the four poles in roughly equal numbers so that each of the four daughter cells receives an approximately normal chromosome number. It is only the combination of chromosomes in these four cells that is faulty; thus, despite a normal chromosome number, they could harbour a combination that leads to the formation of a malignant tumour. To begin with, a more extensive series of counts in different tumours might prove useful. If it should turn out that an exactly diploid chromosome number was regularly found, then our hypothesis must be false [60].

Moreover, chromosome counts within the one tumour would be of importance in that very variable numbers in perfectly healthy tissue or within a homogeneous tumour would weigh against our hypothesis. On the other hand, if there were variable chromosome numbers in the same tumour and these were associated with extensive cell degeneration, especially in those regions where the chromosome numbers are smallest, this would be a finding in support of our hypothesis.

The approach that I myself took, fruitless so far, was to induce multipolar mitoses in healthy tissues in the gentlest way possible and see whether an occasional malignant tumour might be produced in these circumstances. The experiments were carried out in the corneal epithelium and lens epithelium of the rabbit. The procedure was as follows. I destroyed a patch of epithelium, which provoked vigorous mitotic division in the surrounding cells. When this was at its peak, I tried in various ways to inhibit cells that were in the process of dividing. After some time, I destroyed another patch of tissue in order, where possible, to induce renewed division in the tetraploid cells produced by the earlier suppression of cell division – hopefully, simultaneous tetrapolar division. Since the experiments were fruitless I shall not go into them any further. But I do not see the lack of success so far as an argument against my hypothesis. In the first place, in my view, one's initial expectation would be that only a very protracted series of experiments would be meaningful; and, second, the number of multipolar mitoses produced at the right time by the destruction of tissue was much too small to encourage the hope of success.

Now that it has been established that carcinomas can be produced by the action of parasites and, in particular, now that the appearance of sarcomas following transplantation of certain carcinomas comes close to permitting us to speak of the experimental production of malignant tumours, our hypothesis can be tested in a way that is the opposite of what I have just described. If, as

60. The correct diploid chromosome number in man was not established until 1956, 42 years after the publication of Boveri's monograph. Argument still rages about whether there are any strictly euploid carcinomas.

Bashford has found, there are strains of mouse carcinoma that, on transplantation, systematically produce a sarcoma within a period of 6 weeks, it should be possible to determine the time of onset of this new malignancy with tolerable accuracy. If, at that time, abnormal mitoses are especially abundant in the connective tissue adjacent to the transplanted carcinoma, this would support our hypothesis, whereas the absence of such abnormal divisions or of abnormal nuclear events in general would make our hypothesis untenable.

There are still many other facts to be gleaned from the histological and experimental study of malignant tumours and from clinical and statistical evidence that could provide criteria for the validation of our point of view. I have mentioned many of them in Chapter IV. For in this field, as in any other, many important phenomena remain unobserved despite the most assiduous investigation because they are not anticipated by any of our current concepts and must therefore appear to be adventitious concomitants.

If, finally, I may be permitted to send this essay off with a wish, it is that those engaged in research on malignant tumours might be persuaded by my arguments to look at the results they have so far obtained from the point of view set out here and ask themselves in their future studies whether what they find out contradicts my hypothesis or lends it support.

References

AICHEL, O. (1911) Über Zellverschmelzungen mit qualitativ abnormer Chromosomenverteilung als Ursachen der Geschwulstbildung. [Concerning cell fusion together with abnormal chromosome division as causes of tumour formation.] Vorträge u. Aufsätze über Entwicklungsmechanik. Engelmann, Leipzig

BALTZER, F. (1910) Über die Beziehung zwischen dem Chromatin und der Entwicklungs- und Vererbungsrichtung bei Echinodermenbastarden. [Concerning the relationship between the chromatin and the course of development and inheritance in interspecific crosses in echinoderms.] Arch. f. Zellforschung, Bd. 5

BOVERI, T. (1902) Über mehrpolige Mitosen als Mittel zur Analyse des Zellkerns. [Concerning multipolar mitoses as a means of analysing the cell nucleus.] C. Kabitzch, Würzburg and Verh. d. phys. med. Ges. zu Würzburg. N.F., Bd. 35

BOVERI, T. (1907) Zellenstudien. VI. Eine für die erste Orientierung geeignete Darstellung dieser und anderer Chromosomenprobleme findet sich in meiner Schrift: Ergebnisse über die Konstitution der chromatischen Substanz des Zellkerns. [Cell Studies. VI. An introductory treatment of this and other chromosome problems can be found in my article: Findings concerning the constitution of the chromatic substance of the cell nucleus.] Jena 1904

CHILD, C.N. (1907) Amitosis as a factor in normal and regulatory growth. Anat. Anz., Bd. 30

HEIDENHAIN, M. (1894) Neue Untersuchungen über die Zentralkörper usw. [New investigations on the centrosome, etc.] Arch. f. mikr. Anat., Bd. 43

81

HERBST, C. (1900) Über das Auseinandergehen von Furchungs-
und Gewebezellen in kalkfreiem Medium. [Concerning the
separation of primary blastomeres and tissue cells in calcium-
free medium.] Arch. f. Entw. Mech., Bd. 9

HERTWIG, O. AND HERTWIG, R. (1887) Über den Befruchtungs-
und Teilungsvorgang des tierischen Eies unter dem Einfluss
äusserer Agenzien. [Concerning the fertilization and subsequent
division of the animal egg under the influence of external agents.]
Jena

HERTWIG, O. (1910, 1911, 1912) Sitzungsberichte der K. preuss.
Akademie der Wiss

JUSELIUS, E. (1910) Experimentelle Untersuchungen über
die Regeneration des Epithels der Cornea usw. [Experimental
investigations concerning the regeneration of the epithelium
of the cornea, etc.] Arch. f. Ophthalmologie, Bd. 75

KAUTZSCH, G. (1912) Studien über Entwicklungsanomalien bei
Ascaris. [Studies on anomalies of development in Ascaris.]
I. Arch. f. Zellforschung, Bd. 8

WINIWARTER, H. VON (1912) Études sur la Spermatogenèse
humaine. [Studies on human spermatogenesis.] Arch. de
Biologie, T.27

WOODRUFF, L.L. (1913) Dreitausend und dreihundert
Generationen von Paramaecium ohne Konjugation oder
künstliche Reizung. [Three thousand three hundred generations
of Paramaecium without conjugation or artificial stimulation.]
Biolog. Zentralblatt, Bd. 33. No 1

NOTES